A

LECTURE NOTES ON
Forensic Medicine

LECTURE NOTES ON
Forensic Medicine

D. J. GEE
M.B. B.S. M.R.C.Path. D.M.J.

Professor of Forensic Medicine
University of Leeds

SECOND EDITION

BLACKWELL SCIENTIFIC PUBLICATIONS
OXFORD LONDON EDINBURGH MELBOURNE

© 1968, 1975 BLACKWELL SCIENTIFIC PUBLICATIONS
Osney Mead, Oxford,
85 Marylebone High Street, London W1M 3RA,
9 Forrest Road, Edinburgh,
P.O. Box 9, North Balwyn, Victoria, Australia

ISBN 0 632 00257 3

FIRST PUBLISHED 1968
SECOND EDITION 1975

Distributed in the United States of America by
J. B. Lippincott Company, Philadelphia
and in Canada by
J. B. Lippincott Company of Canada Ltd, Toronto

Printed in Great Britain by
WESTERN PRINTING SERVICES LTD, BRISTOL
and bound by
THE KEMP HALL BINDERY, OXFORD

To Eileen

Contents

PART THREE
Toxicology

Introduction

This book is intended to provide the undergraduate with an account of the basic principles of the subject so as to equip him with sufficient knowledge to be able to recognise and cope with minor medico-legal problems arising in his practice and to appreciate when he needs further information and specialised assistance. Detail, therefore, especially in the field of toxicology, is omitted. Further information can be obtained from any of the textbooks listed on p. x. The advent of a second edition has enabled me to incorporate many of the helpful suggestions of reviewers of the first edition.

The plan and presentation of the subject matter are based on the content of the courses of lectures in Forensic Medicine in the University of Leeds, originally developed by Professor C. J. Polson. I express my thanks to him for many years of wise counsel, and to numerous other colleagues for all their assistance. My gratitude to another is expressed elsewhere.

Textbooks for Reference or Further Reading

CAMPS F. E. and CAMERON J. M. (1971). *Practical Forensic Medicine*. Hutchinson, London.

Glaister's Medical Jurisprudence and Toxicology (1973). Ed. Rentoul and Smith. Churchill Livingstone, London.

Gradwohl's Legal Medicine. Ed. Camps (1968). 2nd Ed. Wright, Bristol.

LOCKET S. (1957). *Clinical Toxicology*. Henry Kimpton, London.

MATTHEW H. and LAWTON A. A. H. (1972). *Treatment of Common Acute Poisonings*. Churchill Livingstone, London.

POLSON C. J., BRITTAIN R. P. and MARSHALL T. K. *Disposal of the Dead*. (New Ed. in press.)

POLSON C. J. and GEE D. J. (1973). *The Essentials of Forensic Medicine*. Pergamon Press, Oxford.

POLSON C. J. and TATTERSALL R. N. (1969). *Clinical Toxicology*. The English Universities Press Ltd, London.

SIMPSON K. (1962). *Doctor's Guide to Court*. Butterworths, London.

SIMPSON K. (1965). *Taylor's Principles and Practice of Forensic Medicine*, 12th Ed. J. and A. Churchill Ltd, London.

SIMPSON K. (1974). *Forensic Medicine*, 7th Ed. Edward Arnold, London.

PART ONE

Medico-Legal Aspects of Medical Practice

CHAPTER 1

The Medical Profession and the General Medical Council

A member of the medical profession has been trained in the practice of medicine, has demonstrated his competence by passing a qualifying examination, and is bound by a code of conduct to protect the interests of his patients. Therefore it is necessary that members of the public may be able to distinguish a practitioner with these qualifications from an unqualified person who, although practising medicine, has not received such a training and is not bound by any code of conduct.

Up to 1858 there were no satisfactory means by which a person in need of medical attention could make such a distinction. The first attempt was made during the reign of Henry VIII by an Act of Parliament which put control of the profession into the hands of the Royal College of Physicians, and gave the College powers to prosecute unqualified practitioners. This failed to suppress quacks.

The main statutory regulations establishing the medical profession were made in the nineteenth century. The most important Acts are:

Medical Act 1858

This Act had the stated object of distinguishing qualified from unqualified medical practitioners. A governing body for the profession, the General Council, was established, with duties to compile and maintain a Medical Register, to supervise medical education, and to exercise disciplinary functions. At this time practitioners could qualify for

3

inclusion in the Register on grounds of experience, even though not possessing qualifying diplomas. Penalties were incurred by persons falsely pretending to be registered.

Medical Act 1886

This made possession of a qualifying degree or diploma obligatory before registration. The General Council was made responsible for maintaining the standard of such qualifying examinations. Provision was made for election of some members of the Council by the registered practitioners; previously the Council had only consisted of persons nominated by the Crown, and representatives of the various licensing bodies, i.e. the Colleges and Universities granting degrees or diplomas recognised as registrable qualifications. The Act also made provision for the recognition of medical qualifications of Colonial (now Commonwealth) countries.

Medical Act 1950

This Act made a period of postgraduate training under supervision compulsory, during which time the practitioner is provisionally registered. Proof of having completed such training satisfactorily is necessary before full registration. The General Medical Council became officially so called, and a committee of its members, called the Disciplinary Committee, was formed to enquire into alleged instances of unprofessional conduct, a function which had previously been exercised by the whole Council. The maximum penalty for falsely purporting to be a fully registered medical practitioner was raised by this Act to £500.

Medical Act 1956

This amended and consolidated the previous statutes.

Medical Act 1969

Various modifications of the register were introduced, with two lists of registered persons, the *principal* list, and the *overseas* list, and with a separate register for *temporarily* registered doctors. Provisionally registered, Commonwealth and foreign practitioners are to be indicated in the register. In addition to the initial registration fee, the G.M.C. was empowered to charge an annual retention fee. The term 'serious professional misconduct' replaced 'infamous conduct', and the G.M.C. may suspend a doctor's registration as an alternature to erasure.

General Medical Council

Constitution

At present the Council consists of 47 members: 8, including 3 lay members, nominated by the Privy Council; 11 who are elected by members of the medical profession; and 28 who represent the various licensing bodies, i.e. the Royal Colleges and the Universities.

Functions

Education. The Council is responsible to Parliament for maintaining a standard of proficiency among members of the profession. This is done by:
Requiring Medical Schools and Examining Bodies to submit particulars of their courses of study and examinations.
Appointing Visitors of Medical Schools and Inspectors of Examinations.
Making recommendations regarding the Medical Curriculum.

The Medical Register. This is compiled by the Registrar of the Council and is published annually. It contains the

names, qualifications, dates of registration and addresses of
all provisionally and fully registered medical practitioners.
The qualifying degree or diploma and various approved
additional qualifications may be registered. The entry in
the Medical Register is accepted by the Courts as proof of
the doctor's status. A list of registered medical practitioners
residing overseas is also kept, and may be published as 'the
Overseas Medical Register'. An additional register is kept
of *temporarily registered practitioners*, that is doctors holding a recognised Commonwealth or foreign qualification
and accepted for employment restricted to a hospital or
institution approved by the Council.

Registration allows the doctor certain privileges. He is
entitled to use the description 'registered' or 'duly qualified
medical practitioner'. He may hold appointments in most
hospitals and public services, practise within the National
Health Service, issue certain statutory certificates, such
as death certificates, and prescribe controlled drugs. He can
sue for fees unless he is a Fellow of the Royal College of
Physicians. He may be exempted on application from jury
service. Provisional registration restricts the doctor to
practise within hospital in certain approved training posts,
but within these posts he may practise as though fully
registered.

The Medical Register is kept up to date by means of
periodic enquiries by post to registered practitioners, asking
them to confirm that the entry under their names in the
Register is correct, e.g. that there has been no change of
address.

Removal of a practitioner's name from the Register may
occur in certain circumstances:

1   On the death of the practitioner. This event will be
notified to the G.M.C. by the Registrar of Births and
Deaths.

2   Penal erasure (see below).

3   Failure to reply to the Registrar's enquiry.

4   Failure to pay the annual retention fee.

5 Entries made by error or fraud.
6 On the request of the practitioner, at the discretion of the General Medical Council.

Discipline. By law the G.M.C. is given disciplinary jurisdiction over registered medical practitioners, but only to the extent of deciding whether a doctor has been guilty of conduct which renders him unfit to remain a member of the profession. Therefore the only punitive action which the Council may take is to remove the name of the doctor from the Medical Register thereby indicating that he is no longer a member of the profession. It does not impose fines or other forms of punishment.

Circumstances leading to disciplinary enquiry. (1) *Conviction of a statutory offence*—The conviction of a doctor of any offence in a Court of Law, whether grave, e.g. rape, or trivial, e.g. a driving offence, is automatically notified to the G.M.C. by the Clerk of the Court. The finding of adultery by a doctor in a Matrimonial Court will also be notified.

(2) *Accusation of serious professional misconduct* (this term has replaced the older form 'infamous conduct')—Such a complaint may be brought by a member of the public or a fellow-practitioner or a person acting in a public capacity. The allegation concerns conduct which is not a statutory offence, but may constitute a breach of medical ethics.

A definition of infamous conduct was given by Lopes, L.J., in 1894, viz:
'If a medical man in the pursuit of his profession has done something with regard to it which would be reasonably regarded as disgraceful or dishonourable by his professional brethren of good repute and competency, then it is open to the G.M.C., if that be shown, to say that he has been guilty of infamous conduct in a professional respect.'

Examples of serious professional misconduct

A comprehensive list of types of behaviour which would constitute infamous conduct does not exist. The G.M.C. has
never consented to express an opinion on a hypothetical
situation. Therefore it is only possible, by way of warning,
to give examples of conduct which have, in the past, been
judged infamous, and which had led to penal erasure after
disciplinary enquiry.

In an examination emergency the student would probably
be able to remember the oft-quoted five A's:
Abortion
Adultery
Advertising
Addiction
Association

To supplement the following fuller list, the pamphlets
issued by the G.M.C. on professional discipline should be
consulted.

Abuse of doctor's knowledge, skill or privileges. (a) *Illegal
abortion*—This is one of the most heinous of all medical
sins, and a doctor who is shown to have been guilty of such
action is almost certain to be 'struck off'. Therefore it is
particularly important that a doctor should avoid even
suspicion of this offence. If he is consulted by a pregnant
woman, and there appears to him to be adequate medical
reasons, physical or psychological, for the termination of
the pregnancy, he should always refer the case to recognised
specialists in the relevant fields of medicine, and obtain their
opinions, before embarking on any course of action (see
Therapeutic Abortion, Chapter 4).

Moreover, he should be scrupulously careful to avoid
being implicated unknowingly in the procuring of an abortion. He should be quite sure of the nature of any minor
gynaecological operation or procedure at which he is asked
to assist, or administer an anaesthetic.

He should also be very wary of performing a gynaeco-logical examination in his surgery, when witnesses are absent, on a woman of child-bearing age, lest she is pregnant, and having subsequently aborted, accuses him of being responsible. Indeed, if the woman should die of some complication of the abortion, he might be charged with manslaughter.

(b) *Improper use of controlled drugs*—This means the use of drugs to produce or gratify addiction, either of the doctor or his patient. It also covers the commission of offences contrary to the Misuse of Drugs Act, for instance the purveying of such drugs to unauthorised persons.

Therefore it again behoves the doctor to avoid any possible suspicion by understanding and adhering strictly to the relevant law, e.g. by ensuring that his supplies of controlled drugs are accurately accounted for. He should be especially cautious when prescribing drugs of addiction, particularly to young people with non-fatal illnesses, and to temporary patients, who may be addicts, using a story of absence from their usual medical practitioner as a means of obtaining supplies of drugs; over-prescription must be avoided, and drugs not used by a patient must be retrieved and destroyed, lest they are disposed of to unauthorised persons.

Abuse of the doctor-patient relationship. (a) *Adultery or improper conduct or association* with a person with whom the doctor has a professional relationship constitutes infamous conduct.

The professional relationship may be obvious, as when the person concerned is the doctor's patient, or less immediately apparent, as when the person is a relation of a patient. The important point is that the doctor made the acquaintance of the person as the result of his professional services, and that the adultery or improper association commenced while the professional relationship existed, even though it was subsequently severed.

An improper relationship may exist, short of actual

adultery. Thus the following comments were made by the Judicial Committee of the Privy Council, when upholding a decision of the Disciplinary Committee. 'A doctor gains entry to the home in the trust that he will take care of the physical and mental health of the family. He must not abuse his professional position so as, by act or word, to impair in the least the confidence and security which should subsist between husband and wife. His association with the wife becomes improper when by look, touch, or gesture he shows undue affection for her, when he seeks opportunities of meeting her alone, or does anything else to show that he thinks more of her than he should. Even if she sets her cap at him, he must in no way respond or encourage her. If she seeks opportunities of meeting him, which are not necessary for professional reasons, he must be on his guard. He must shun any association with her altogether, rather than let it become improper. He must be above suspicion.

'It was suggested that a doctor, who started as the family doctor might be in a different position when he became a family friend. His conduct on social occasions was to be regarded differently from his conduct on professional occasions. There must, it was said, be cogent evidence to show that he abused his professional relationship. This looks very like a suggestion that he might do in the drawing-room that which he might not do in the surgery. No such distinction can be permitted. A medical man who gains the entry into the family confidence by virtue of his professional position must maintain the same high standard when he becomes the family friend.'

(b) *Improper disclosure of confidential information*—This matter is discussed in Chapter 7. Briefly, a doctor should normally keep secret any information obtained about his patients, and only divulge it on direction of a Judge in a Court of Law. On the occasions when it becomes necessary, in the interests of the community, for the doctor to disclose knowledge obtained in confidence, he must observe the rules of privileged communication.

Disregard of responsibilities to patients. (a) *Gross negligence in diagnosis or treatment*—The subject of negligence is dealt with in Chapter 6. To constitute infamous conduct the doctor's actions would have to go beyond the sphere of ordinary negligence on one occasion, even though that would render the doctor liable to civil action, and would have to consist of persistent and gross neglect of his patients' interests by failing to apply accepted methods of diagnosis and treatment, as a result of which the patients were harmed. Persistent failure to attend patients through idleness or carelessness would constitute such conduct.

(b) *Covering*—This means associating with unregistered medical practitioners in such a way that members of the public are misled as to their true status. Thus, by administering anaesthetics to enable such a practitioner to perform operations, the doctor might cause patients to believe that the operator himself was a member of the medical profession, or that his methods had received general approval by the profession. Allowing such a person to use the doctor's premises, staff, or instruments might have the same effect.

Personal tendencies dangerous to patients. Alcoholism and drug addiction—A doctor who suffers from either of these conditions is obviously liable to be a danger to his patients, and is unfit to continue in practice. However they are curable, and so when a complaint or a notification of conviction is received for the first time in respect of a particular doctor, the Disciplinary Committee of the G.M.C. may postpone its decision in order to allow the doctor time to undergo treatment. Nevertheless alcoholism or drug addiction constitutes serious professional misconduct, and repeated complaints or notifications of conviction, e.g. for drunken driving, will result in penal erasure.

Conduct discreditable to the doctor, or to the profession. This will principally arise from evidence, e.g. by notification of conviction, that a doctor has been guilty of such offences as fraud, forgery, theft, etc.

False or misleading certificates. As the number of forms or certificates to be completed during the course of medical practice continues to increase, so does the risk that a doctor, from overwork or carelessness, will be tempted to issue them without ensuring that the information he gives is accurate. But he does this at his peril. To issue a National Insurance Certificate without seeing the patient, or to complete cremation form C while confined to bed by illness, without having seen the body or the doctor issuing form B, is to invite criticism, or worse, disciplinary proceedings, and deliberate falsification of certificates is a very serious offence.

Profiting at the expense of his colleagues. (a) *Canvassing*— Although it is perfectly normal in commerce for a business man to send circulars to potential clients indicating in laudatory terms the value and scope of his services, such behaviour on the part of a doctor would constitute infamous conduct. Neither should he attempt to attract another doctor's patients to his own practice by word of mouth, or any other means.

It is, of course, permissible to inform patients on the doctor's own list of a change in the doctor's address or telephone number, but such notification should be confined to a simple statement of the alteration, and should be sent in an envelope to ensure that it is only seen by the person for whom it was intended.

(b) *Advertising*—The blatant forms of advertising such as advertisements or articles in the lay press drawing attention to a doctor's abilities, or large and elaborate signs at his surgery are obvious and fortunately rare.

More difficult problems arise in the fields of broadcasting and the writing of books and articles intended to be read by the general public, and in lecturing to lay audiences. To remain anonymous is usually the best safeguard against accusations of advertising, at the same time ensuring that nothing said or written by the doctor could be interpreted as being directed towards his own personal advantage.

(c) *Deprecation of other doctors*—Whether criticism of another doctor is justified or not, it should never be made in the presence of patients or members of the public. If a doctor feels that one of his colleagues is deserving of censure, his correct course is to inform the G.M.C.

Abuse of financial opportunities. Examples of such abuse are:

Improperly obtaining money by demanding fees from Health Service patients when they are entitled under the National Health Service Acts to free treatment.

Commercialisation of a secret remedy.

Dichotomy or 'fee-splitting' as when part of a private patient's fee is handed by a specialist to the general practitioner as a reward for having referred the patient to him.

Prescribing drugs or appliances in which the practitioner has a financial interest. This, of course, would only apply to undue prescribing when the doctor had a considerable financial interest, e.g. was a director of a company. It does not refer to the doctor who holds a few shares in some drug company.

Disciplinary procedure

Notifications of convictions of doctors and complaints of their misconduct are received by the Registrar and submitted by him to the President. Trivial matters may be dismissed at this stage. Otherwise the complaint or conviction is then considered by a small committee, the Penal Cases Committee.

Penal Cases Committee

This consists of the President and five other members, one of whom is a layman. Its function is to make preliminary enquiry into the case, in order to decide whether it merits investigation by the Disciplinary Committee.

Allegations of professional misconduct must be supported by a statutory declaration, unless the allegation is made by a person acting in a public capacity, e.g. an officer of a Government Department or a local authority. The doctor concerned is invited to submit an explanation of his conduct for consideration by the Committee.

The Committee may refer the case to the Disciplinary Committee, may send a warning letter to the doctor in the case of the first conviction of an offence such as drunken driving, or may consider that no action is necessary.

Disciplinary Committee

This Committee consists of 19 members, 2 of whom are laymen, but usually only 9 members sit at a hearing. No member of this Committee other than the President may also be a member of the Penal Cases Committee.

The procedure of the Committee is similar to that of a Court of Law. The accused practitioner is notified of the date of the hearing not less than 28 days beforehand, and is informed of the nature of the accusation. He is entitled to be legally represented. Witnesses may be subpoenaed to attend and give evidence on oath.

If the Committee is considering the conviction of a doctor (in a Court of Law), it is bound to accept the fact of conviction as proof that the doctor was guilty of the offence charged. Similarly the finding in a matrimonial court of adultery by a doctor is proof of the fact. The Committee's purpose in such a case is to decide whether the nature of the offence or conduct merits erasure of the doctor's name from the Register. In cases of alleged infamous conduct evidence may be called before the Committee from either side to determine the truth of the allegation.

Having considered the facts the Committee may receive evidence in mitigation from the accused doctor. It then has to decide whether the facts justify erasure of the doctor's name from the Medical Register, or suspension of his registration for a period of up to 12 months. There is no other form of punishment, but a form of probation exists, whereby the Committee may postpone its decision for a stated interval, e.g. 6 months, at which time the facts are reconsidered and evidence of the doctor's behaviour during the interval is produced, before a final decision is made. This course of action may be deemed appropriate, for instance, in cases of alcoholism, or drug addiction, by giving time for the doctor to undergo treatment.

Appeals

The doctor whose name is to be erased or suspended may appeal to the Judicial Committee of the Privy Council against the decision of the G.M.C. Such an appeal must be lodged within 28 days of the decision.

Restoration after erasure

A doctor whose name has been erased from the Register after disciplinary proceedings may apply to have his name restored at any time after 10 months from the date of erasure, and if unsuccessful at intervals of 11 months thereafter. Such restoration is not unusual if evidence of satisfactory behaviour subsequent to erasure is available, and the original offence was not too grave.

Summary of Disciplinary Procedure

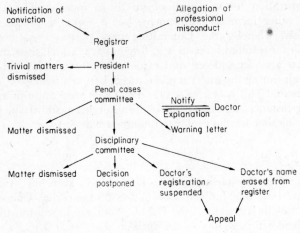

Fig. 1

CHAPTER 2
Certification of Death and Disposal Procedure

The legal procedure, following a death, may be summarised as follows:

1   The cause of death must be ascertained and certified by death certificate or determined by Coroner's investigation.

2   Details of the death and of the deceased are recorded by the Registrar of Births and Deaths.

3   The body must be disposed of, by any lawful means, normally burial or cremation.

Notification of cause of death

Death certificate

Regulations for the issue of death certificates have existed since 1874. The object of the certificates is to prevent the concealment of crime, and to obtain information, for statistical purposes, of causes of death in the population.

1   *When may a doctor issue a death certificate?*
(a)   If he is a registered medical practitioner.
(b)   If he attended the deceased during the last illness.

In practice this usually means where the doctor attended within 14 days of the death. In some cases when the doctor was attending the deceased regularly *and had seen the body after death*, the certificate may be accepted even though the last attendance was more than 14 days before death. A practitioner who sees the deceased for the first time after death, such as a locum, or a partner of the usual medical attendant, is not entitled to issue a certificate.

(c)   *If he knows the cause of death.* According to the law, if the two previous criteria are satisfied the doctor must always issue a certificate, even if the cause is unknown or obviously unnatural. The Registrar would then notify the Coroner. However, the usual practice in such cases is for the doctor to notify the Coroner himself, and withhold the certificate.

2   *The form of the certificate*
The certificate must be in the form prescribed by the Registrar General and books of such certificates, together with the franked envelopes for their dispatch, can be obtained from the local Registrar of Births and Deaths.

The Death Certificate is reproduced by courtesy of HMSO.

Note

1   The doctor is not at present obliged to see the body after death before issuing the certificate. It is advisable to do so, however, in case the death has resulted from some injury sustained since the doctor last visited, or lest death has not in fact occurred.

2   When stating the cause of death, precise terms of the responsible morbid conditions, e.g. cerebral haemorrhage or coronary thrombosis, should be used. Vague terms, such as asphyxia or heart failure, are not acceptable. The book of certificates contains a list of undesirable terms. If the terminal event is a consequence of pre-existing diseases, these must be recorded in the correct sequence, e.g.

	Ia	Cerebral haemorrhage
due to	Ib	Hypertension
due to	Ic	Chronic nephritis

Any other condition independently contributing to death, but not forming part of the sequence, should be noted in Part II

e.g.   II   Chronic bronchitis

Examples of correct certification are given in the book of certificates for the guidance of doctors.

3   If any of the conditions listed in parts I or II may have an unnatural cause, the Registrar will refer the case to the Coroner. Therefore ambiguous terms such as 'gangrene' or 'cirrhosis' should be qualified by an indication of the cause, e.g. cardiac cirrhosis or alcoholic cirrhosis.

4   The spaces A and B on the reverse of the form are likely to be rarely used. The doctor should initial A when he has both notified the Coroner and also issued a death certificate, a practice which is strictly correct but hardly ever followed. Space B should be initialled if he is awaiting the results of some laboratory investigation, e.g. a swab culture, which may provide additional information of value for statistical purposes.

5 The qualifications which the doctor appends must only be those entered in the Medical Register.

6 Certification is to the best of the doctor's belief and knowledge. Subsequent demonstration that his diagnosis was incorrect does not make him guilty of an offence. Nevertheless, he must use the utmost care in completing the certificate.

7 On completion of the certificate the doctor retains a counterfoil, sends the certificate to the Registrar, and detaches and hands the Notice to Informant (see below) to the appropriate person.

8 The certificate is a statutory document, i.e. required under the Births and Deaths Registration Act. No fee may be charged by the doctor, but he may be prosecuted for failing to issue a certificate if he is eligible to do so.

The Informant

This is the person whose duty it is to register the death. Usually he is a relative of the deceased, but the back of the Notice to Informant bears a list of people who may be required to act if no relative is available, e.g. the person causing the disposal of the body. The informant must take the Notice to the Registrar, and register the death within 5 days.

Still-Birth Certificate

By law any registered medical practitioner or certified midwife who was present at a still-birth, or examines the body of a still-born child must give to the person qualified to act as informant for the purpose of registration, a certificate of still-birth, in the prescribed form.

If the informant cannot for any reason obtain such a certificate he may make a statutory declaration of still-birth to the Registrar and explain why the certificate is not available. This anachronism is unlikely to be used nowadays.

B

The definition of a still-born child is a child which has been born after the twenty-eighth week of pregnancy and which did not, after having been completely expelled from its mother, breathe or show any other sign of life. Signs of life, in addition to breathing, are movement, heart-beat, or pulsation of the umbilical cord.

As in the case of death certificates, still-birth certificates are obtainable from the Registrar of Births and Deaths in book form.

Note

1 In stating the cause of death, indefinite terms must be avoided. (Examples are given in the book of certificates.) The nomenclature of the International Classification of Causes of Still-birth should be used.

2 If the doctor was not present at the birth, he should be very cautious before forming an opinion of still-birth on external examination of the body, unless some obvious congenital malformation incompatible with life, or maceration of the body, is present. Any uncertainty is best resolved by reference to the Coroner.

3 There is a counterfoil to the certificate, but no Notice to Informant. The doctor hands the completed certificate to the informant instead of sending it to the Registrar.

4 The informant may be: the mother; the father of a legitimate child; a person present at the birth; the occupier of the house in which the birth occurred.

5 The still-birth must be registered within 42 days and the birth must be notified to the Medical Officer of Health.

Notification of a death to the Coroner

The doctor has no statutory duty to notify any death to the Coroner. He complies with the law if he issues a death certificate, even though the death is due to an unnatural cause, and leaves the Registrar to inform the Coroner. There is, however, a duty in Common Law for every person 'about a body' to notify the Coroner of circumstances likely to require the holding of an inquest, but this duty is not enforceable. The generally accepted practice is for the doctor personally to notify the Coroner of a death and not to issue a death certificate, avoiding thereby much inconvenience and waste of time.

There is no official list to guide the doctor in deciding when to refer a death to the Coroner. A simple rule is to refer all deaths known to be due to unnatural causes, or when the cause is unknown. Examples of the type of death which *should* be referred are as follows:

1   Deaths from violence—accidental, suicidal or homicidal. This applies whether death results immediately and directly from the injury, or is indirectly related, after a lapse of weeks, months or even years.
2   Deaths following abortion.
3   Deaths from privation or neglect—including self-neglect.
4   Deaths from poison and alcoholism.
5   Deaths during surgical operation or anaesthesia.
6   Deaths from industrial disease.
7   Deaths of persons in receipt of war pensions.
8   Deaths from unknown causes.

(For the procedure of Coroner's Investigations see Ch. 10.)

Registration of death

The informant must attend the Registrar, to give details of the deceased to be entered on the Register, and to hand to the Registrar certain documents, such as the medical card and any papers relating to pensions received by the deceased from National Funds, e.g. war pensions. The Registrar will record the cause of death as given on the death certificate. He has a statutory obligation to inform the Coroner of deaths in certain circumstances, as when the cause of death

---

The Still-birth Certificate is reproduced by courtesy of HMSO.

appears to have been unnatural, or if the deceased had not been attended by a medical practitioner during his last illness. Death certificates containing ambiguous terms which might indicate an unnatural cause, e.g. cirrhosis of the liver, will undoubtedly cause the death to be referred to the Coroner.

If the Registrar is satisfied that there is no need for further enquiry into the death, he will authorise disposal of the body by issuing a certificate for Disposal after Registry. Disposal of a body without authorisation from the Registrar or the Coroner is illegal.

Procedure in Scotland and Eire

In Scotland a death certificate may be issued by a doctor who knows the cause of death, even if he was not in attendance during the last illness. Deaths from unnatural or unknown cause are referred to the Procurator Fiscal, who takes the place of the English Coroner. The death certificate is different in form, and has no notice to informant. It must be delivered to the Registrar within 7 days of the death.

In Eire, under the provisions of the Coroner's Act of 1962, a medical practitioner must notify the Coroner of the death of a patient whom he has not attended during the preceding month, or whom he knows to have died of one of a list of specified conditions.

Disposal of the body

Burial

The Registrar's Certificate for disposal is delivered to the person arranging the funeral, e.g. the undertaker. After burial a notification of disposal is sent by the undertaker to the Registrar.

The duty to arrange for disposal of the body is usually

that of the executor, or the next of kin of an intestate. The Local Authority must act if no-one else is available, e.g. in the case of a person without relatives. Under the National Insurance Act, 1946, a Death Grant is provided to cover the cost of disposal.

Cremation

First a medical certificate of cause of death must be issued, the death must be registered and the Registrar's certificate for disposal must be obtained. In addition application must be made to the cremation authorities for cremation of the body, by submission of several different forms. The more stringent regulations applied to this method of disposal are designed to ensure that evidence of crime is not destroyed, and that cremation is not carried out against the wishes of the deceased or a relative.

Form A. The application for cremation, submitted by the person having the duty to dispose of the body. Any objections to cremation known to have been made by the deceased or any relative and any reason to believe that death was due to violence, poison, or neglect, or that a further examination of the body is necessary must be stated. The form is countersigned by a person in authority, e.g. an M.P., or a police officer, who knows the applicant.

Form B. A medical certificate given by the doctor who issued the death certificate. Details are required of the mode of dying as well as the cause of death, and the doctor must have examined the body after death. He must disclose any relationship he had to the deceased, and any pecuniary interest which he may have in the death.

Form C. A confirmatory medical certificate given by a practitioner of at least 5 years' registration. He must not be related to the deceased or to the doctor issuing form B. He also must examine the body after death, and see and question the doctor giving form B.

Both doctors must state that they have no reason to believe that the death was due to any unnatural cause, or that any further examination of the body is necessary.

Form F. The authority to cremate. It is issued by the medical referee of the cremation authority (who is usually also the local M.O.H.) after scrutiny of the previous forms, when he is satisfied that all requirements of the cremation regulations have been fulfilled.

After cremation a certificate of disposal is sent to the Registrar, as in the case of burial.

Special forms

Form D. A certificate of cause of death issued after a post-mortem examination, ordered or performed by the medical referee when he has considered further investigation of the cause of death to be necessary. It replaces forms B and C, but is rarely used in England and Wales.

Form E. The Coroner's certificate of cause of death, issued after a post-mortem examination has been made at his direction, or an inquest has been held. It replaces the medical certificates on forms B and C, but not form F. It is not the authority to cremate.

Disposal in special circumstances

Anatomical dissection

The procedure to be followed, as laid down by the Anatomy Acts, is complicated. If a patient expresses a wish that his body should be used for dissection, the doctor should advise him to contact the local teacher of anatomy, e.g. the Professor of Anatomy in a medical school, who will supply the relevant forms, and explain the procedure. If the patient merely indicates his wishes in his will, and no arrangements are made before his death, difficulties are likely to arise.

Disposal of parts of a body—Human Tissue Act 1961

This Act makes lawful the removal of tissues of a deceased person for therapeutic purposes and for medical education and research. It replaced the Corneal Grafting Act of 1952. It also permits the performance of post-mortem examinations to establish or confirm the cause of death, provided that the death is not one which should be notified to the Coroner.

Removal of tissues. Tissues may be removed if the deceased requested this in writing at any time, or orally during his last illness in the presence of two or more witnesses.

If no such request had been made, the person lawfully in possession of the body, i.e. the hospital management committee or board of governors, may authorise the removal of tissues provided that there is no reason to believe after reasonable enquiry that the deceased had expressed an objection to such a procedure, and that the surviving spouse or relatives do not object.

Removal must be by a fully registered medical practitioner who has satisfied himself that life is extinct. No tissues must be removed if there is reason to think that the death should be reported to the Coroner.

Recently modifications of this procedure have been proposed, in Bills put before Parliament, to allow a medical practitioner to authorise removal of organs if the deceased has registered his consent in a register maintained by the Secretary of State.

Post-mortem examinations. Such an examination may be

authorised by the person lawfully in possession of the body, provided that:

1   The Coroner does not require to investigate the death.

2   Reasonable enquiry has shown that the deceased or any surviving relative has not objected.

Such examinations may be performed by a fully registered medical practitioner or, on his instructions, by a provisionally registered practitioner or medical student.

Exhumation

This may be to allow removal of a body to another burial ground, and authorisation is then given by the ecclesiastical authorities. Exhumation for other reasons is normally authorised by a licence from the Home Office or may be by a Coroner's Order. This may occur, for instance, when a death which has been certified as being due to natural causes appears on subsequent information to have been due to poisoning.

Dying declarations

On occasions a patient dying as a result of a criminal act may yet be able to make a statement about the events, which will be able to be used at any subsequent trial, and the doctor should assist the person to give such evidence. However, certain rules must be obeyed for the statement to be valid.

1   The patient must be aware that he is dying, and that *he has no hope of recovery*, and must state this in the declaration.

2   The precise words of the patient must be recorded, if possible in writing at the time and signed by the patient, though an oral statement may be acceptable, recorded in writing as soon as practicable.

3   The patient must not be suffering from mental confusion.

4   The matter of the statement must only concern the

circumstances responsible for the patient's approaching death.

Dying depositions

If a person is dangerously ill and unlikely to recover, a magistrate may take evidence on oath from him, and such a deposition may be used subsequently at a trial as evidence, if the patient has died or is too ill ever to attend court. Since there is opportunity for full cross-examination the deposition may relate to subjects other than the cause of the patient's illness or death.

CHAPTER 3
Medico-Legal Aspects of Mental Disease

The purpose of this chapter is to outline the legal provisions for safeguarding the person and property of people suffering from mental disorder, or protecting the public, and to indicate how a person's disordered mental state may affect his responsibility under civil and criminal law. It does not deal with the clinical aspects of psychiatry.

Before 1890 there were few legal provisions for safeguarding the interests of mentally ill persons. The Lunacy Act of 1890, which was the principal Act until 1959, established, among other things, the procedure for compulsory admission of patients to mental hospitals after examination by a Justice of the Peace, if the patient was certified as being of unsound mind by a medical practitioner.

Provision for voluntary admission of a patient was first made by the Mental Treatment Act of 1930.

Mental Health Act 1959

This Act replaced the older statutes, in the light of the modern views on the medical treatment of mental illness. Only certain parts of the Act are considered here. For full details the Act itself or the various pamphlets issued by the Ministry of Health should be consulted.

Classification of mental disorder

The Act defines certain classes of mental disorder. These are important since they affect the provisions made for patients.

Mental disorder—mental illness, arrested or incomplete development of the mind, psychopathic disorder, and any other disorder or disability of mind.

Severe subnormality—a state of arrested or incomplete development of mind which includes subnormality of intelligence and is of such a nature or degree that the patient is incapable of living an independent life or guarding himself against serious exploitation.

Subnormality—a state of arrested or incomplete development of mind (not amounting to severe subnormality) which includes subnormality of intelligence and is of a nature or degree which requires or is susceptible to medical treatment or other special care or training of the patient.

Psychopathic disorder—a persistent disorder or disability of mind (whether or not including subnormality of intelligence) which results in abnormally aggressive or seriously irresponsible conduct on the part of the patient, and requires or is susceptible to medical treatment.

Admission to hospital

Voluntary Admission. This is intended to be the principal means by which patients shall be admitted, wherever possible.

Compulsory Admission. These provisions are only intended to be used when no other method is applicable and the patient constitutes a danger to himself or others.

(i) *Admission for observation.* A patient may be compulsorily admitted for observation for a period not exceeding 28 days. The application may be made by the nearest relative or the Mental Welfare Officer, who must have seen the patient within 14 days prior to the application. The Mental Welfare Officer, whose old title was 'Duly Authorised Officer', may be contacted through the Mental Health section of the Local Health Authority (Sect. 25).

The application must be supported by written recommendations of two doctors, one of whom must have special experience of mental disorder, while the other will usually be the patient's regular medical attendant. The recommendations need not indicate the precise nature of the mental disorder, but must state that compulsory detention is necessary in the interests of the patient, or others. The recommendaions must be given before the application is made, and neither doctor may make the application himself, or be related to the applicant. During the 28 days the patient may be discharged, or admitted for treatment either voluntarily or compulsorily.

(ii) *Admission for treatment.* Such an application may be made in respect of a patient of any age suffering from mental illness or severe subnormality, but only for those suffering from subnormality or psychopathic disorder, if they are under the age of 21 years (Sect. 26).

The applicant may be the nearest relative or the Mental Welfare Officer, but the latter may not make such application if the nearest relative objects.

Two medical recommendations are required, as in the case of admission for observation, but in this case they must specify the nature of the illness, on which they must be in agreement, and indicate that other methods of treatment are not suitable.

Admission is initially for 1 year, and may be renewed for a further year, and then at 2-yearly intervals.

(iii) *Admission for observation in an emergency.* In such a case application may be made by any relative, or by the Mental Welfare Officer. It is supported by one medical recommendation, usually by the regular medical attendant. The applicant must have seen the patient within 3 days prior to making the application (Sect. 29).

Such an emergency admission may only last for 72 hours, but during this time the formalities may be completed for admission for observation for 28 days.

Provisions also exist (Sect. 136) for removal of a mentally-ill person by a police officer to a 'place of safety', such as a mental hospital, where the person may be detained for up to 72 hours.

Compulsory reception into guardianship

Guardianship means the care of a patient, outside hospital, by some person or, more usually, the local authority. The guardian has powers in relation to the patient equivalent to those of a parent over a child under the age of 14 years.

Applications are in general similar to those for compulsory admission to hospital, and must be supported by two medical recommendations. Such application may not be made for persons suffering from subnormality or psychopathic disorder, who are over the age of 21. The patient under guardianship must be visited regularly by a nominated medical practitioner. The guardianship is initially for

1 year, and may be renewed as in the case of admission to hospital for treatment.

Discharge of patients

An order for discharge of a patient may be made by the hospital or local authorities, and may also be made by the nearest relative in cases of admission for treatment, or for guardianship. The relative ordering discharge must give 72 hours' notice to the authorities, and discharge may be prevented if during this time the responsible medical officer makes a report stating that the patient would be likely to behave dangerously if discharged.

In the case of patients suffering from subnormality or psychopathic disorder, the provisions of guardianship cease to apply after they have reached the age of 25 years; nor may they be compulsorily detained in hospital after this age unless a medical report indicates that they would be likely to be dangerous to themselves or others if released.

Leave of absence

Patients under compulsory detention may be granted leave of absence by a responsible medical officer. If absent without leave they may be taken into custody and returned to the hospital, by any mental welfare officer, officer of the hospital, or constable, unless they have been absent for more than 28 days, or in the case of subnormal or psychopathic patients over the age of 21, for more than 6 months.

Mental health review tribunals

These are appointed for each Regional Hospital Area by the Lord Chancellor. The members are chosen from the legal profession, the medical profession, or are persons having experience of administrative or social welfare work. A tribunal must contain one member from each of these groups.

The function of the Tribunal is to consider appeals against guardianship or compulsory detention in hospital from patients or relatives, and it may direct the discharge of a patient whom it considers is not suffering from mental illness at the present, or if further detention is considered to be unnecessary.

Provision for mentally ill patients charged with criminal offences (Sects. 60, 61 and 65)

Compulsory admission to hospital or guardianship. A Magistrate's Court or a Crown Court (previously Assizes), on convicting a person of any offence other than murder, may order his compulsory admission to hospital or guardianship if:

1   Oral or written evidence of two doctors, one of whom has special experience of mental disorder, shows that the offender is suffering from mental illness, psychopathic disorder, subnormality or severe subnormality of a nature or degree which warrants the detention of the patient.

2   In the circumstances such detention is the best method of dealing with the case.

3   A hospital or guardian can receive the person.

A patient who has been admitted to hospital or guardianship on a court order is treated as though he has been compulsorily admitted for treatment, or received into guardianship in the usual way, except that his discharge may not be ordered by the nearest relative, and the special provisions for expiration of authority in respect of persons suffering from psychopathic disorder and subnormality will not apply. On appeal the Mental Health Review Tribunal may order the patient's discharge.

Court order restricting discharge of the patient. Such an order may be made by a Crown Court (previously Assizes), if it is considered necessary for the protection of the public. Before such an order is made at least one doctor must give oral evidence relating to the offender's mental state.

A magistrate's court may not impose such an order. If it seems necessary to restrict the patient's discharge, the case must be referred to a higher court.

If such an order is imposed only the Home Secretary may authorise leave of absence or the discharge of the patient. The patient may ask that his case be referred by the Home Secretary to the Mental Health Review Tribunal.

Care of a mental patient's property

A court known as the Court of Protection exists for this purpose, with a Master and Deputy Master who are appointed by the Lord Chancellor. A judge of the court, having heard medical evidence to show that a patient's mental state prevents him from managing his own affairs, may make such directions as are necessary to control the patient's property or carry on his business, or, more commonly, may appoint a receiver to attend to such matters.

The court can authorise the execution of a will on the patient's behalf; it will then require medical proof that the patient lacks testamentary capacity.

Certain legal and medical practitioners, who are appointed by the Lord Chancellor and are known as the Lord Chancellor's Visitors, have the responsibility of visiting such patients periodically and reporting to the judge on the patient's ability to manage his own affairs. The medical Visitor may require to examine the patient or to see any medical documents relating to the case, which may be in the possession of the patient's usual medical attendants.

Civil responsibility of mental patients

Contracts

A contract which has been entered into may be binding on

the parties even though one party suffers from mental illness, unless it can be shown that the patient was incapable
of understanding the contract and the other party knew of
his mental illness, i.e. had perpetrated a fraud.

Torts, i.e. civil wrongs

A person is held to be responsible for his actions provided
that he knows their nature and quality, and in such a case
may be sued for damages.

Marriage

In the contract of marriage mental illness may be a ground
for declaring the marriage null, or for divorce (see Chapter
4).

Witness

A person, even though suffering from mental illness, may
be considered capable of giving valid evidence if the Court
decides that the person is capable of understanding the
significance of the oath and the necessity of telling the truth,
and can make a coherent statement of the facts of a matter.

Making a will—testamentary capacity

A doctor may be required to examine a person suffering
from mental disorder who wishes to make a will, in order
to ascertain whether his mental state will permit a reasoned
disposal of his property. Subsequently the doctor may be
required to give evidence in court if the will is contested. A
doctor would be well advised not to witness a patient's will
unless he is prepared to testify later to the person's testamentary capacity, and as a witness he will forgo any legacy
which he might have received from the will.

In deciding the capacity of the patient to make a will, the points which the doctor should consider are:

1   Does the patient realise he is making a will?
2   Does he know what property he possesses?
3   Does he understand which people have reasonable grounds for benefiting by the will?
4   Does he suffer from delusions which will cause unreasonable decisions?

Criminal responsibility of mental patients

If a person has committed a crime, notably homicide, his responsibility for his act, and the punishment to which he may be liable, can be modified to varying degree by the existence of mental illness, either at the time of the act or afterwards, e.g.:

Not guilty by reason of insanity

This is the modern version of the old verdict of 'Guilty but insane', amended by the Criminal Justice Act 1948. It is based on the M'Naghten Rules of 1843, which were framed by a panel of judges after the trial of a man who, while suffering from a mental illness, shot and killed the secretary of Sir Robert Peel. Basically these state:

1   Every man is presumed sane and responsible for his acts until the contrary is proved.
2   To establish the defence it must be proved that at the time of the act the accused, by reason of disease of the mind, did not know what he was doing, or if he knew what he was doing then he did not know that it was wrong.

Diminished responsibility

This defence was established by the Homicide Act 1957, to cover those cases where, although the accused was not insane to a degree necessary to come within the M'Naghten

Rules, yet his mental responsibility for his act was substantially impaired by some abnormality of mind, such as arrested or retarded development or conditions caused by disease or injury.

In such a case, the accused's action in killing another is reduced from murder to manslaughter.

Other cases

Unfit to plead. If an accused is sent for trial at a Crown Court the defence may attempt to prove that the prisoner is suffering from mental disturbance to the extent of being unfit to be tried. This is based on medical evidence that the prisoner is unable to understand the nature of the evidence, to instruct his counsel or to follow the procedure of the trial. If the jury is satisfied on these points the prisoner, without standing trial, will be sent to Broadmoor or some other mental hospital.

Insane after conviction. If a patient is considered to be insane after he has been convicted of an offence, he may be dealt with under the appropriate sections of the Mental Health Act 1959, or the Home Secretary may order a special enquiry into the prisoner's mental state.

CHAPTER 4
Medico-Legal Aspects of Marriage, Divorce and Disputed Paternity

Impotence

This is the inability of a person to satisfy sexual desire in another, i.e. to have sexual intercourse, and may constitute a ground for nullity of marriage. It is not the same as sterility; a person may be unable to have children but may be quite capable of achieving sexual intercourse.

Impotence may be temporary or permanent, and may be due to age, general or local illness, or deformity of the sexual organs. Medical examination to determine the presence of such a condition may be required in cases of nullity of marriage or alleged rape.

Sterility

This does not constitute grounds for nullity of marriage or divorce.

Sterilisation by means of voluntary vasectomy is now legal (National Health Service, Family Planning Amendment Act 1972).

Artificial insemination by a donor (A.I.D.) has recently received the sanction of the B.M.A.

Nullity

A marriage may be declared null and void by the Courts on various grounds. Basically these show that either (a) one or other of the persons was incapable of being a party to a contract, e.g. from mental disorder, or (b) had in effect perpetrated a fraud, e.g. by being pregnant by someone else at the time of the marriage, or by being incapable of ever carrying out the requirements of the marriage contract, as by being impotent.

The principal grounds for a declaration of nullity of marriage are as follows:

1 Incapacity, or impotence. This is when the marriage cannot be consummated, i.e. it is impossible for there to be full penetration of the vagina by the penis, either from physical or mental disease, or deformity which cannot be corrected. Doctors will be required by the Court to examine

both the husband and the wife to determine whether there
is in fact any bar to the consummation of the marriage.

2   If one or other party deliberately refuses to consum-
mate the marriage. Obstinacy, hysteria, frigidity, vaginis-
mus, etc., may cause such a situation.

3   If a person, at the time of their marriage, was suffering from mental disorder so as to render them unfit for
marriage, or was suffering from recurrent attacks of insanity
or epilepsy.

4   If one of the parties was, at the time of the marriage,
suffering from venereal disease in a communicable form.

5   When the wife, at the time of the marriage, was pregnant by a man other than the husband.

If a decree of nullity is sought on the grounds mentioned
in paragraphs 3, 4 or 5 above, the petitioner must have
been ignorant of the facts at the time of marriage, must
institute proceedings within a year of the marriage, and
must not have consented to marital intercourse since dis-
covering the facts.

A marriage may also be declared void because of some
'administrative irregularity' such as the existence of a prior
marriage of one of the parties, marriage within the prohibited degrees etc. These matters are not likely to require
medical evidence.

Divorce

The sole ground for a petition for divorce, under the
Divorce Reform Act 1969, is that the marriage has broken
down irretrievably.

Proof of breakdown of the marriage may be that:

(a)   the respondent has committed adultery and the
petitioner finds it intolerable to live with the respondent.

Adultery occurs when one of the parties has voluntary
sexual intercourse with someone other than the spouse. The
doctor is rarely required, or indeed is able, by physical
examination to prove that a married person has had extra-

marital intercourse. However, it may be alleged that a child born to the wife could not have been fathered by the husband. The grounds for such an allegation may be that the duration of pregnancy indicates that conception must have occurred at a time when the husband could not have had intercourse with the wife, e.g. if he was in another country. Alternatively, blood group determination may show that the husband could not be the father of the child (see below).

(b) the respondent has behaved in such a way that the petitioner cannot reasonably be expected to live with the respondent.

This corresponds to the old grounds for divorce of 'cruelty'. A doctor may be required to give evidence of injuries inflicted on the petitioner before the divorce proceedings were commenced, or to interpret injuries to general health, such as insomnia or weight loss.

(c) the respondent has deserted the petitioner for a continuous period of at least two years immediately preceding the presentation of the petition.

(d) the married couple have lived apart continuously for 2 years and both parties agree to the divorce.

(e) the couple have lived apart for a continuous period of at least 5 years.

The last three matters are unlikely to involve a doctor, except in the case of mental illness of one of the parties.

Pregnancy

It may be important on certain occasions for the Courts to have medical evidence that a woman is pregnant, though a woman cannot be compelled to submit to examination for such a purpose.

1 A woman convicted of a capital offence. Formerly pregnancy constituted a bar to execution, though of course it is exceedingly unlikely that any woman will be in danger of execution in the future.

2 The fact that a woman is pregnant may affect the

disposal of property by a will, since the unborn child may have a claim on the estate.

3 In cases of alleged abortion or concealment of birth, or in cases of libel or slander, where a woman has been accused of illicit sexual intercourse. Actions for breach of promise no longer exist, and so a doctor should beware becoming involved in such disputes.

Signs of pregnancy

These are all dealt with in textbooks of obstetrics. To summarise, they are:

1 Presumptive—
   Cessation of menstruation
   Morning sickness
   Breast changes
   Abdominal enlargement
   Hegar's sign
   Uterine contractions
2 Conclusive—
   Foetal movements
   Foetal heart sounds
   X-ray demonstration of foetal structures
   Biological tests

Period of gestation

This may be of importance in cases of alleged adultery. The normal period is approximately 280 days, or 40 weeks. Living children can of course be born at 6 or 7 months of gestation, though they are then obviously immature. Conversely, a pregnancy may be protracted, and since courts are loath to pronounce a child illegitimate, durations of pregnancy of 331 days and up to 349 days have been accepted, but a duration of 360 days rejected.

Where a husband is shown to have had access to his wife, i.e. has been able to have sexual intercourse with her, as by being in the same house, and the child is born after a reasonable subsequent period of gestation, it will be taken to be his child, by the Courts, unless illegitimacy can be proved by some other means, such as blood group determination.

Delivery

Medical evidence of recent delivery in a person may be sought in cases of alleged abortion or infanticide, or concealment of birth, and in disputed legitimacy of an offspring, e.g. when it is alleged that a woman has 'borrowed' an infant, and has pretended to have given birth to it, in order to gain some financial or social benefit, by fraud.

Signs of recent delivery are only summarised here, but details should be sought in obstetric textbooks.

1   Breast changes—production of milk.

2   Abdominal striae gravidarum.

3   Enlargement of uterus, softening of cervix, recent damage to perineum. Lochia.

4   Biological pregnancy tests.

Disputed paternity

This may arise in various circumstances, e.g.

1   A married man may allege that his wife has committed adultery, and that he is not the father of a child which she has borne.

2   An unmarried girl who has an illegitimate offspring may allege that a certain man is the father of the child, in order to obtain an affiliation order against him.

In either event, the Court may seek medical assistance in determining the paternity of the child.

Such evidence may be called regarding the duration of pregnancy, as to whether it is consistent with conception having occurred at a time when the husband had access to his wife.

On occasions proof of parentage may be accepted on the grounds of close physical resemblance of the child to the alleged father, but such resemblance would have to be striking, such as distinctive colouring, or the presence in both parent and child of an obvious congenital deformity such as a supernumerary digit.

The use of blood group determination as a means of excluding a certain person as the parent of the child has a more reliable scientific basis, and is becoming increasingly used in the Courts; under the provisions of the Family Law Reform Act 1969, a court may direct that blood tests be used, if one of the parties to the proceedings applies. Samples of blood cannot be taken from any person without consent, but in the case of refusal the court may draw the appropriate inference.

Blood group determination

The various human blood groups are known to be factors which are inherited on the lines established by Mendelian principles. Thus they provide a means of indicating the possible parentage of a child, since they are inherited characters which are easily determined.

The basic facts which make the blood groups of value in this field are (a) that a person's blood group remains constant throughout his life, except for transient disturbances after transfusion, and (b) that a person's blood group must be inherited from his parents, so that he cannot have a blood group which is not possessed by either of his parents (except in the very rare event of a spontaneous mutation).

On Mendelian principles a person inherits one gene for each blood group from each parent, who themselves may be homo- or heterozygous for the particular group. Thus in a blood group with several factors the result may be complicated. The principles may be demonstrated by considering the ABO group, e.g.:

		Group
(a)	Mother	A (genotype AO)
	Child	O

Possible fathers 1. B (genotype BO)
                       2. A (genotype AO)
                       3. O
                       4. AB impossible—no O gene

(b)	Mother	A
	Child	AB

Possible fathers 1. B or AB possible
                       2. A impossible—no B gene
                       3. O impossible—no B gene

The same principles may be used for other blood group systems, of which the most commonly used after the ABO system are the Rhesus and the MNS systems, following the same general principles.

Blood grouping cannot identify any particular person as the father of a child. Thus grouping may show that the child's father must be Group B, but will not show which of the many people possessing Group B blood. On the other hand the blood grouping may serve to exclude one particular person as the father, and this exclusion is the value of the method. The chance of exclusion of a person who is not the father is 30% using the ABO system. Obviously the more blood group systems which are tested independently then the greater the chance of exclusion, e.g. the best chance of an innocent man being excluded at the present is about 60%, calculated from the gene frequencies of the various blood groups.

Taking the blood samples

Regulations under the Family Law Reform Act give details of how blood samples should be taken. A direction form as specified in the Regulations is sent to the doctor by the Court.

There is provision in the form for a photograph of the person from whom the Court has directed the sample to be taken, a declaration that the subject has not received a blood transfusion recently and forms of consent from the subject, or, if the subject is under a disability (e.g. a young child), the person having care of the subject. The form of the report of the person making the blood tests is also specified, and a scale of fees laid down.

Sufficient blood may be obtained from an infant by a heel prick, but it is preferable to delay the testing of the infant until it has reached the age of 1 year, as before this time the agglutinins (Anti-A and Anti-B) will not have developed.

Therapeutic abortion

The termination of pregnancy on medical grounds has become lawful, subject to the provisions of the Abortion Act 1967. Before the enactment of this statute, medical practitioners acting in good faith had to rely for protection from prosecution on decisions made in the Courts, notably R. v. Bourne 1936, which established precedents but were not binding on other Courts.

The main provisions of the Abortion Act are:

That termination of pregnancy is lawful when carried out by a registered medical practitioner, provided that two registered medical practitioners are of the opinion, formed in good faith:

1 that the continuance of the pregnancy would involve risk to the life of the pregnant woman or of injury to the physical or mental health of the pregnant woman or any existing children in her family greater than if the pregnancy were terminated; or

2 that there is a substantial risk that if the child were born it would suffer from such physical or mental abnormalities as to be seriously handicapped;

3 in determining whether the continuance of a pregnancy would involve such risk of injury to health as is

mentioned in paragraph (1) account may be taken of the pregnant woman's actual or reasonably foreseeable environment.

Termination must be carried out in a Health Service Hospital, or a hospital approved for this purpose by the Minister of Health or the Secretary of State.

A registered medical practitioner may terminate a pregnancy, even though the opinion of two registered medical practitioners is not available and the termination is not to be performed in a Health Service or approved hospital, provided that in the particular case he is of the opinion, formed in good faith, that the termination is immediately necessary to save the life or to prevent grave permanent injury to the physical or mental health of the pregnant woman.

No person can be compelled to participate in any treatment authorised by this Act, if he has a conscientious objection; but this does not affect a duty to participate in treatment which is necessary to save the life or prevent grave permanent injury to the physical or mental health of a pregnant woman.

CHAPTER 5
Consent

A doctor does not have an automatic right to submit anyone to a medical examination or treatment. A physical examination, if conducted without the consent of the patient, could constitute in law (a) a criminal offence, an assault, either common or indecent, depending on the type of examination, or (b) a trespass upon the person. Therefore, it is important that the doctor should understand the different forms of consent, and also the circumstances in which each would be appropriate.

Occasions when consent not required

(a) On admission to H.M. Prison—for routine examination.
(b) On a court order, of a person suffering from a notifiable disease or tuberculosis.
(c) On the probation order of a court.
(d) Of immigrants at ports and airports.
(e) Of milk or food handlers.
(f) Of school children, in state schools.

Thus all these cases are where refusal to allow examination might jeopardise the health of the community as a whole, or a substantial portion of it. In all other cases consent is necessary to medical examination.

Validity of consent

For a person's consent to be valid it must be genuine and freely given. He must understand exactly what he is consenting to, and within reason what any possible results or complications might be. The consent must not be obtained by any sharp practice or blackmail, such as making some action of the doctor dependent on the consent of the person to some other procedure. Consent obtained by force, or fear, or fraud is always invalid.

The fact of consent when appropriate must be clearly stated. The fact that the patient doesn't say no, or obeys without saying anything, does not indicate consent.

It is especially important to remember to ensure that consent is valid when dealing with persons suspected or accused of having committed some criminal offence.

Forms of consent

1 Implied.
2 Express—oral or written.

Implied

i.e. by the behaviour of the patient. Thus the fact that a patient attends the surgery or summons the doctor to his house, complaining of illness, implies that he consents to a general physical examination, to determine the nature of the ailment. This implied consent is sufficient for all normal medical practice, but not if intimate examinations are to be made, e.g. rectal or vaginal examinations.

Express

i.e. specifically stated by the patient either orally or in writing.

Oral consent—where possible this should be given in the presence of a third party, otherwise the doctor has no proof of its existence if subsequently challenged. Oral consent should be sought before any of the intimate examinations, rectal or vaginal, before the performance of procedures such as a gastric test meal, or the taking of blood samples. A third person who is a disinterested party, i.e. not a friend or relative of the patient, should be present when an intimate examination is made to protect the doctor from subsequent accusations of indecent assault.

Written consent—this is necessary for the major procedures such as the administration of anaesthetics or the performance of operations. It is also necessary for examinations of persons accused of criminal offences. The protection societies have indicated the ideal consent form to be used in hospital, which makes it clear that the nature of the procedure and any complications have been explained to the patient, who also understands that the procedure is not to be carried out by any particular doctor.

Valid consent cannot be obtained for a procedure which is illegal, such as euthanasia.

Consent in special cases

Normally consent as described above is given by the person concerned. However, this may not be possible, or may need to be qualified.

By a spouse

In operations interfering with marital rights, such as abortion or sterilisation, the consent of the patient is paramount, but the consent of the spouse should also be sought, though this cannot override the wishes of the patient. If the patient is unconscious or otherwise unable to give valid consent, then the consent of the spouse will be valid.

Minors

Under 16 years of age. The consent of the parent or guardian is necessary. If neither is available then the consent of the person in *loco parentis*, e.g. the headmaster of the child's school, is valid, in an emergency.

On occasion parents may refuse permission for a procedure on their child which is necessary to save life, on religious grounds, e.g. blood transfusion is objectionable to Jehovah's Witnesses. It is possible then for a magistrate's court to order the child's removal from the care of the parents to that of a 'fit person', e.g. a county welfare officer, who may then give valid consent. However the Minister of Health has advised hospitals against adopting this procedure. Even if the doctor acts without consent, in such circumstances, provided that he does so in good faith to preserve the child's life, then he is unlikely to be in danger of legal action.

Over 16 years of age. Such a person can give valid consent, even though not yet 18. However, it is advisable to consult parents if practicable.

Consent in emergency

If the patient is unconscious and no-one is available who could give consent, the doctor is entitled to carry out any procedures necessary to preserve life, but no more. Thus he may give blood transfusions, perform operations to relieve raised intra-cranial tension, etc. But a badly damaged limb, for instance, should not be amputated, provided that it does not constitute a danger to life, even if there is no doubt that subsequently it will be useless, without first obtaining the patient's consent.

CHAPTER 6
Negligence

Any citizen can be guilty of negligence. For a person to be judged negligent:
1   He must owe a duty to another person.
2   He must have committed a breach of that duty.
3   As a result the person to whom the duty was owed must have suffered some damage.

Translating this into terms of medical practice:
1   The person must be the doctor's patient, i.e. someone for whose medical care the doctor accepts responsibility.

2 The doctor must have done something which is not approved medical practice, or, more commonly, have omitted to do something which is considered accepted practice in the circumstances.

3 As a result of the action or omission the patient has suffered injury.

For example—a person attends casualty and is seen by the Casualty Officer (who accepts responsibility). He has suffered a fall on the hand which is painful, but no X-ray is taken and therefore no fracture diagnosed (omission of approved medical practice). Due to malunion of the fracture arthritis develops with incapacity of that hand (the patient has suffered damage).

When is duty owed?

This is from the moment that the doctor undertakes advice or treatment, whether under contract or gratuitously, e.g. at the scene of an accident. The doctor has no legal obligation to undertake the care of any patient, but once the obligation is accepted then he is liable to exercise proper skill and care in the management of the case.

Standard of duty

No doctor is expected to be perfect or infallible. The standard of competence which the patient is entitled to expect is that of an ordinary competent practitioner in the grade or speciality to which the doctor belongs. Thus the degree of skill expected in any one field of medicine is that of the average practitioner in that field. But a doctor would be ill-advised to go outside his sphere of competence. Thus a general practitioner performing major surgery will be expected to exercise the degree of skill of an average surgeon, unless he was forced to act in an emergency, when no surgeon was available.

Breaches of duty

Approved practice

If a doctor has followed approved medical practice, this will be taken as evidence of due care. Departure from approved practice, e.g. failure to take X-rays or to give ATS in appropriate circumstances, is risky, leaving the doctor little defence if anything goes wrong. Doctors are expected to keep reasonably up to date by reading medical journals, but no-one is expected to read all the journals and be aware of all advances.

Accurate diagnosis

No doctor guarantees accuracy of diagnosis, and therefore cannot be considered negligent if an inaccurate diagnosis is made, unless it is shown that he did not exercise proper care in making it, e.g. failure to examine the abdomen of a child suffering from appendicitis, or failure to keep the child under observation if such a condition were suspected.

Risks of treatment

Some risks are inherent in any form of treatment and the doctor will not be negligent if they cause damage provided that he has taken reasonable care to avoid them, e.g. broken needle during injection. However, he may be negligent if he doesn't warn the patient beforehand of any appreciable risk involved, or inform him after a mishap has occurred.

Thus a needle would not be anticipated to break, and the patient need not be warned of the possibility. However, if it has broken then the patient should be told and arrangements made to remove the broken piece. If the doctor fails to notice that the needle has broken, or, having discovered this, does not tell the patient or make arrangements to prevent further damage, then he is negligent.

C

Communication with other doctors

Failure to inform a general practitioner of a person's discharge from hospital and treatment might constitute negligence if there was a reasonable possibility of some complication of the condition occurring. It has been held that such communication must be direct. To advise the patient to attend his own doctor or to give him a verbal message for the doctor in such circumstances is insufficient. This applies more to emergency treatment.

Attendance on patients

Failure to attend a private or Health Service patient promptly when called may be held negligent when due to forgetfulness or laziness.

Res ipsa loquitor. This is a legal term meaning 'the thing speaks for itself'. Thus if after an operation the patient is found to have a swab or a pair of forceps left in the abdomen, this cannot be considered reasonable treatment, and the facts automatically indicate negligence. The onus then shifts to the doctor, to explain the facts if he can, or to show that the negligence was not his.

Criminal Negligence

This is rare, and only occurs if the negligence is so gross that compensation is an inadequate redress and it constitutes a crime deserving punishment. This type of negligence is seen in a grossly careless act which results in death of a patient, as in obstetric delivery while drunk, or administration of an anaesthetic while under the effects of drugs. The doctor will then probably be charged with manslaughter and, upon conviction, may also be struck off the Medical Register.

Medical defence societies

In any question of negligence the doctor would be well advised to consult his medical defence society before taking any action, in particular before making any admission. He should also remember that nowadays disclosure of a patient's medical records can be compelled and so he should be careful to ensure that the records are complete, accurate, and do not contain any derogatory comments, exposure of which could be embarrassing for him.

CHAPTER 7
Professional Secrecy—Privileged Occasions

Normally a person is responsible for his statements and their consequences and may be sued for slander or libel, i.e. defamation of character. However, there are occasions when it may be necessary for a doctor as a duty to the public to make a statement which is derogatory. Then the doctor's statement is privileged if he acted in accordance with the rules, and he has a complete defence.

Usually any information received by a doctor from a patient is confidential and may not be disclosed to any other person. However its disclosure may be compelled in a court of law, even when treatment is given under a promise of secrecy, e.g. for venereal disease.

Absolute privilege

This applies to any statements made in Parliament or in a court of law. No one can be sued over any statements made in these places.

Qualified privilege

This provides protection against legal action when persons make statements in the course of their legal or social duty, but only if certain rules are observed:

1   The statement must not be malicious.
2   It must only be made to those having an interest or duty to receive it.

For example the statement on a death certificate that a person has suffered from syphilis is privileged, but the same statement made in conversation to a general member of the public is not protected and may result in legal action. Or, if a person is suffering from an infectious disease the doctor may need to inform the patient's employer, and would be protected against subsequent legal action, but not if the statement was also made to the patient's workmates.

Thus a doctor must be very careful, when making statements about a patient, to whom he makes the statements.

Secrecy

At times there may be a difficult conflict between a doctor's duty to respect the confidence of his patient and to divulge information for the benefit of the community. Thus in the case of a motorist who is found to suffer epileptic attacks, it may be necessary to inform his employer or works medical officer, if the patient refuses to disclose the facts himself. However regulations now permit the issue of a driving licence to an epileptic who has had no fits during the day for 3 years. Pregnancy in a girl under 16 years needs to be disclosed to the parents, but over 16 the girl's consent must be obtained first. A doctor was accused, though aquitted, of infamous conduct for disclosing to her parents that a girl of 16 had been prescribed contraceptive pills by a clinic.

In the case of a road traffic accident the law obliges a doctor to divulge information to the police, but generally the doctor should observe secrecy.

CHAPTER 8
Compensation

A person who suffers an injury as the result of an accident will usually be able to claim compensation. This may be by legal action in a civil court against the person responsible for the accident, or it may be a claim on the State under the National Insurance Acts.

In either event, a doctor is likely to be required to give evidence of the nature and consequences of the patient's injuries, and their relationship to the accident.

Medical precautions

It is as well for a doctor to remember that any injury which he is called upon to treat may later become the subject of a claim for compensation, and that such a claim, especially where civil law action is involved, may take a year or more before the stage is reached where the doctor's evidence is required. A legal control, under the Limitation Acts, is imposed to prevent unreasonable delay in commencing legal action for compensation for a personal injury. Such an action must usually be started within 3 years from the date

of the injury, unless the injury is of a type which is only
slowly manifested. In such a case the claimant must show
that material facts of a decisive character relating to his
injury were unknown to him until 3 years had elapsed, and
that the action was started within 12 months of the discovery of those facts, and the leave of the court must be
obtained. Even so by the time the legal procedure has
reached the stage of a court hearing a doctor may find himself giving evidence about an event which occurred 4 or 5
years previously.

Therefore whenever he treats an injury, however trivial,
he should remember the possibility of litigation at some time
in the future, and should be particularly careful to make
adequate notes of the nature of the injury and the treatment given and whether the patient's disability was or was
not related to the accident. These he can refer to when
called upon to give evidence many months later. If the
injury is of any magnitude, and requires prolonged treatment, then the notes should contain assessments of the
amount of pain, distress, etc. involved, since these may need
to be considered later when a Court is assessing damages,
and can only be estimated reliably by the doctor. Loss of
earnings, and the impairment of abilities at the time of the
claim can usually be assessed by the Court without the
doctor's help, but he may be required to express an opinion
as to the prognosis of any disability.

It is, of course, well known that conditions may be attri-
buted by the patient to an injury, but without any founda-
tion in fact. Also the degree of a person's disability may be
considerably exaggerated by psychological disturbances of
the patient, i.e. compensation neurosis, the condition being
alleviated by settlement of the claim in the patient's favour.
This is not the same as malingering, where the person
deliberately falsifies symptoms and injuries for gain, financial or otherwise, but in either case the doctor must be
ready to detect and take into account these conditions when
giving opinions about the patient's disabilities.

In addition to treatment of a living patient, the doctor may be required to decide whether a person's death was a consequence of an accident or injury, or attributable to his work, since the dependants may then have grounds for claiming compensation.

Relationship between trauma and disease

There are certain conditions which are well-recognised as being consequences of trauma, e.g. pulmonary embolism. There are others where the relationship is very debatable, and is usually denied, e.g. tumour formation, except in a few special circumstances. There is no doubt that this field of Forensic Medicine causes greater dispute than any other. Therefore it is important that the doctor should be cautious, should consider the facts very carefully before expressing an opinion, and should not diverge from accepted medical views unless he has very good reason. Carelessly considered opinions may lead to useless litigation, and to the doctor's discredit and embarrassment.

Examples of certain commonly queried relationships are given here, but obviously the list is by no means exhaustive, since the question of the relation between trauma and almost every known disease could be and probably has been raised.

Conditions commonly accepted as being a sequence to trauma

Venous thrombosis and Pulmonary embolism

Deep vein thrombosis, especially in the legs, possibly associated with pulmonary embolism, is well-recognised as being related to an injury, if it occurs 1 to 2 weeks later, and following a period of immobility. Increased viscosity of the blood, platelet adhesiveness and venous stasis have been suggested as the predisposing factors.

Broncho-pneumonia

This commonly occurs in elderly people following a fracture with consequent immobility; the shock and the immobility with bad postural drainage are the probable causes.

Peptic ulcer

As an acute duodenal ulcer, known as Curling's ulcer, this may occur as a complication of burns or scalds, or of fractures; the mechanism is unknown.

Tumour

In the vast majority of cases it is considered that there is no reason for connecting trauma and tumour development. Experimental work has not revealed any tumour growth after a single injury. However, in a few instances, notably when considering meningiomas, the growth has been found to develop at the exact site of a cranial injury, especially with a fractured skull, as shown by Cushing; the mechanism may be sequestration of fragments of dura in the fracture line. Skin cancer is well recognised as a hazard of radiation. On other occasions, tumours, e.g. of bone, may occur within a few weeks or months of trauma, and in the absence of definite proof to the contrary, a Court is likely to take the view that it is probable that trauma has played a part either in initiating or accelerating the rate of growth of the tumour.

Conditions which may be aggravated by trauma

Coronary occlusion by atheroma

Sudden increased demands for blood by a heart with a deficient arterial supply due to coronary atherosclerosis, may precipitate a cardiac infarction with severe pain, or sudden collapse and death during the exertion. A coronary thrombosis, on the other hand, is rarely related to trauma, except in the uncommon instance when trauma to the chest causes damage to the coronary vessel, which is then followed by thrombosis.

Rupture of aneurysms

Direct violence may occasionally cause rupture of an aneurysm, as for example when a forcible blow to the head causes sub-arachnoid haemorrhage from rupture of a 'berry' aneurysm of a cerebral artery. More commonly the rupture is held to be due to a rise in blood-pressure which is a consequence of unaccustomed physical exertion.

Ewing's postulates

This set of criteria was suggested when considering the relationship between trauma and tumours. However, in general they are applicable in many other situations. It is suggested that in order to establish a probable relationship between an injury and a tumour:

1　The part of the body must have been quite healthy before the accident.

2　It must be proved that adequate trauma was applied to the part.

3　A tumour must have occurred within a reasonable time interval after the trauma.

4　The tumour must occur in the exact location of the trauma.

5　The nature of the tumour must be proved by microscopical examination.

In fact these postulates are an attempt to introduce some rationalism into the common assumption that two events which are closely related in time must be cause and effect. They do not provide very scientific proof of a relationship even when they are satisfied, but by considering them the doctor will often be able to clarify his views on a given situation.

Insurance

Private Insurance

A doctor may be requested by an Insurance Company to make a medical examination of a proposer. It must be remembered that any false information given in a certificate of insurance will cause the policy to be void, and if a doctor deliberately gives false information he may be guilty of fraud and also liable to disciplinary action by the General Medical Council. He must therefore be particularly careful to avoid being persuaded or misled into omitting or ignoring any tests or abnormal findings.

National Insurance

This provides sickness and unemployment insurance for all workers, and retirement pension, widow's pension, maternity grants, etc. Before a claimant can receive many of these benefits a doctor may be required to complete a medical certificate, notably in support of claims for sickness benefit; first, intermediate and final certificates being needed. The doctor should be very careful not to be coerced into issuing such certificates without being satisfied by personal examination that the claimant is in fact sick, i.e. not to issue certificates to a relative wtihout seeing the patient, Such conduct would constitute issuing false certificates, and could lead to disciplinary action by the G.M.C.

Industrial injuries

The National Insurance (Industrial Injuries) Act 1946 replaced the old Workmen's Compensation Acts.

By the provisions of this Act employed persons are insured

by a fund maintained by contributions from the workmen, the employers, and the State, against accidents and certain prescribed diseases occurring at work, or while travelling in connection with work. Such benefit, unlike a civil litigation claim, is payable even though the injured person has disobeyed instructions or safety regulations and had sustained the injury as a consequence. The benefits consist of:

Injury Benefit—during sickness after an accident.

Disablement Benefit—when a permanent disability results.

Death Benefit.

The claimant must:

Give notice of the accident as soon as possible.

Make claims in a standard form.

Submit to a medical examination, and to treatment and rehabilitation, if this is possible.

The Claim, supported by appropriate certificates, goes first to the Insurance Officer. He may allow, or disallow the claim, or may refer it to the Local Appeal Tribunal. The claimant may also appeal to the Tribunal, and after that to the Industrial Injuries Commissioner.

A person claiming disablement benefit is referred by the Insurance Officer to a Medical Board, consisting of two or more medical practitioners who assess his disability. The claimant may appeal against the Board's decision to a Medical Appeal Tribunal.

In addition to accidents, certain diseases, which are recognised as resulting from special forms of employment, are prescribed by the Act and persons in such employment who suffer from them are automatically entitled to benefit.

The diseases and the special forms of employment are listed in schedules to the Act, which should be consulted for full details. Only a few examples are given here.

Schedule Part I

Lead poisoning from any occupation involving the use or

handling of, or exposure to the fumes, dust or vapour of lead or its compounds.

Infection by leptospira icterohaemorrhagiae from work in rat-infested places.

Cataract from the frequent or prolonged exposure to the glare of molten glass or red-hot metal.

Schedule Part II

This defines the occupations responsible for the industrial lung diseases known as pneumoconioses, such as silicosis and asbestosis.

e.g. any occupation involving the dressing of granite or any igneous rock by masons or the crushing of such materials, or substantial exposure to the dust arising from such operations.

Special Pneumoconiosis Boards investigate claims of disability arising from these diseases.

CHAPTER 9
Poisons Legislation

Poisons control

Until recent times the sale of poisons was not subject to any legal control. The first attempt to institute such control was in 1851, when the Arsenic Act was passed. The first comprehensive legislation was the Pharmacy and Poisons Act 1933; the most recent is the Poisons Act 1972.

General control of Poisons

Poisons Act 1972

A panel of experts, known as the Poisons Board assist the Home Secretary to prepare a list of substances which should be considered to be poisons, requiring control; and also to make Poisons Rules, controlling the acquisition, storage, etc., of these substances. The objects of the Rules is to prevent unlawful acquisition of poisons, while at the same time allowing supplies to be obtained by persons having a legitimate reason, with the minimum of inconvenience. The Poisons Rules are revised and consolidated from time to time. The present principal Rules are those of 1972. They can be obtained from H.M. Stationery Office.

Poisons list

This contains all the substances which are considered to require restriction. Some substances which only cause poisoning if taken in large amount, such as aspirin, are not included.

Substances are added to or removed from the list from time to time, on the recommendation of the Poisons Board, and copies of the list may be obtained from the Stationery Office.

The list is divided into two parts:

Part I contains substances used for medicinal purposes; therefore these may only be obtained from authorised sellers of poisons, i.e. registered pharmacists.

Part II contains substances used in industry or agriculture; these may be obtained either from authorised sellers, or from 'listed sellers', i.e. persons whose names are on a local authority list of sellers of Part II poisons, such as proprietors of horticultural shops.

Poison rules

These impose specific restrictions on certain groups of poisons. The rules are divided into 16 schedules, of which only Schedules 1 and 4 are of practical interest to the doctor. The others deal mainly with the manufacture and transport of poisons.

Schedule 1

These rules are concerned with the procedure and recording of the acquisition of certain poisons. These poisons are most of those in Part I of the Poisons List, and a few of those in Part II, and are selected because of their highly toxic nature, being substances which are too dangerous to be freely available to the public. Therefore:

1 These poisons may only be sold under the supervision of a registered pharmacist, on registered premises.

2 The pharmacist must know that the purchaser is a suitable person to be entrusted with the poison. This may be either from personal knowledge, or by a certificate to that effect given by a householder. If the pharmacist doesn't know this householder either, the certificate must be countersigned by a police officer, in charge of a police station.

3 Details of the sale must be recorded in a Poisons Book; the entry must contain the date, name and address of the purchaser, the nature and quantity of the poison, and the purpose for which it is required. The purchaser must sign the entry.

4 A doctor need not attend the pharmacist personally in order to sign the entry in the Poisons Book, by being allowed to send a '*signed order*' bearing the same information as is required for an entry in the Poisons Book. This is then kept by the pharmacist as a record of the transaction.

In an emergency the pharmacist is allowed to supply a poison on a doctor's telephoned instructions but the doctor must furnish a signed order within 24 hours.

5 If a doctor dispenses medicines containing Schedule 1 poisons he must keep records of the amount of poison supplied and to whom, just as the pharmacist does.

6 Poisons in Schedule 1 must be stored separately from foods, and in a cupboard, drawer or shelf reserved for the storage of poisons. Containers must be labelled 'Poison', and bear the name and address of the supplier.

Schedule 4

The rules in this schedule restrict the acquisition of certain drugs to members of the public who hold a prescription given by a registered medical practitioner, dentist or veterinary surgeon.

There are two sections to this schedule, 4a and 4b. The poisons in section (a) are ones which are already controlled by the rules of Schedule 1. Therefore the prescription must be in a precise form since it replaces the entry in the Poisons Book, and is the only record of the sale.

In section (b), the poisons are not controlled by Schedule 1. Therefore the exact form of the prescription is less important.

The pharmacist may supply the poison on telephoned instructions of the doctor, provided that the latter sends a prescription within 24 hours (as with signed orders in Schedule 1).

Section (a). The principal drugs in this part of the schedule are the barbiturates.

The prescription must bear the *name and address of the doctor*, and his signature, the date, the name and address of the patient, the name of the drug, he total amount to be dispensed, and the amount to be taken at each dose.

A prescription given by a dentist or veterinary surgeon must be marked accordingly, e.g. for dental treatment only.

A prescription may be repeated, provided that the number of times it may be repeated and at what intervals is clearly stated. Otherwise, if the doctor omits to indicate how often it may be repeated, the pharmacist may only repeat it three times in all, or if the interval between the repeats is omitted, then it may not be repeated more often than once in every three days. Health Service prescriptions on E.C.10 are not repeated, as the pharmacist retains the prescription.

Section (b). The drugs in this section are mainly those affecting mental states, e.g. tranquillisers and 'stimulants'. The regulations state that these drugs may only be supplied on prescription, but the form of the prescription is not specified, except that it must be dated and bear the doctor's signature. The repetition of prescriptions is controlled in the same way as in section (a).

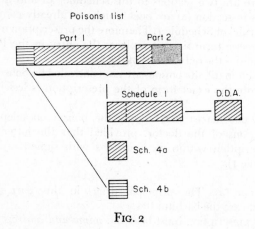

FIG. 2

Control of drug addiction

Previously this was complicated by the number of Acts involved, notably the Dangerous Drugs Acts. Now these have been consolidated and superseded by the Misuse of Drugs Act 1971, which incorporates most of their features.

The Act:

1 Sets up an Advisory Council, charged with keeping under review the situation in the United Kingdom with respect to drugs which are misused (principally drugs of addiction) and advising the Government on measures for their control.

2 The drugs affected by the Act are called 'controlled drugs'. There are 3 classes, e.g.

Class A   (e.g. Morphine)
Class B   (e.g. Cannabis)
Class C   (e.g. Methaqualone)

This classification is concerned with grading penalties for offences when drugs in different classes are involved, e.g. on summary conviction of an offence involving

Class A drug   £400 fine or 12 months imprisonment
Class C drug   £200 fine or 6 months imprisonment

3 It is an offence to import or export controlled drugs, to supply them or to possess them, unless authorised (e.g. a doctor is authorised to possess and supply them).

4 The Home Secretary shall make Regulations, dealing with storage, prescriptions, etc.

5 If a doctor commits an offence under this Act, or if it appears that he has behaved irresponsibly with regard to prescribing or supply, etc., of controlled drugs, or has contravened regulations in respect of supplying or notifying addicts, the Home Secretary may issue a direction prohibiting the doctor from using those or any controlled drugs.

In the event of irresponsible behaviour or contravention of regulations the Home Secretary may refer the case to a tribunal set up under the Act to consider the matter. The tribunal will advise the Home Secretary whether to issue a direction or not. In an urgent case the Home Secretary may issue a temporary direction, after consulting a professional panel, and must then, while the temporary direction is in force, refer the case to a tribunal.

6 If a 'drug problem' appears to be occurring in a particular area, a doctor may be obliged to give details, of controlled

drugs which he has supplied, on the request of the Home Secretary. Details of the patients concerned need not be divulged.

Misuse of Drug Regulations 1973

1 The regulations make an additional classification of drugs, into Schedules, e.g.

Schedule 1   (e.g. codeine)
Schedule 2   (e.g. morphine)
Schedule 3   (e.g. chlorphentamine)
Schedule 4   (e.g. cannabis and L.S.D.)

Anyone can administer drugs in Schedule 1; only doctors or dentists may administer drugs in Schedules 2 and 3.

2   For drugs in Schedules 2, 3 and 4.

(a) *Supply to Doctor.*

This may be by a 'signed order' or requisition in the same form as that described above, under the Poisons Act 1972. In an emergency the doctor may order a supply of drugs by telephone, provided, he supplies a written requisition within 24 hours.

(b) *Prescription.*

Such a prescription may not be dictated by the doctor over the telephone, but in other respects is the same as the form of prescription described above for Schedule 4 (a) drugs under the Poisons Act. However, the doctor, as well as signing and dating the prescription himself, must also *write* the name and address of the patient and the total quantity and dose of the drug. This prevents the issue of prescriptions by unqualified persons such as receptionists.

(c) *Registers.*

For drugs in Schedules 2 and 4 registers must be kept of drugs obtained and of drugs supplied or administered. There must be a separate part for each class of drugs. Entries must be made in chronological order, on the same day that the drug is obtained or supplied, or not later than the next day. The entries must be indelible, and no alteration or obliteration is allowed. The entry must indicate the date, name and address of supplier or person supplied, the authority of a person supplied to possess the drug, the amount of the drug and the form in which it was received or supplied. Loose-leaf books may not be used. If the doctor has more than one surgery, separate sets of records must be kept for each, and these records must be available for inspection at any time for a period up to two years from the date of the last entry.

3 *Safe Custody Regulations.*

These apply to drugs in Schedules 2, 3 and 4. The doctor must keep such drugs in a locked receptacle, which can be opened only by him, or a person authorised by him. A locked car is not a 'locked receptacle'.

4 *Notification of and Supply to Addicts Regulations.*

An addict is defined as a person who, as a result of repeated administration has become so dependent upon the drug that he has an overpowering desire for the administration of it to be continued.

If a doctor attends a person who he diagnoses as a drug addict he must, in the next 7 days, send in writing to the Chief Medical Officer at the Home Office details, e.g. name, address, N.H.S. number. This doesn't apply if the doctor is satisfied that continued administration of drugs is needed for the treatment of organic disease or injury; or notification of the addict has been made within the last 12 months.

A doctor shall not supply to a drug addict any cocaine or heroin, unless he is licensed by the Home Secretary to treat drug addicts, or else the drugs are needed to treat an organic disease or injury.

(For details of drug addiction see Chapter 36).

Control of efficacy of drugs

The Medicines Act 1968, lays down regulations relating to production and dealing in medical products, their sale or supply, clinical trials and advertising.

CHAPTER 10
Court Procedure

Coroner's Court

The office of Coroner is an ancient one; certainly dating from the time of William I, possibly earlier. His original powers and duties were extensive, but today his function is mainly restricted to the investigation of obscure or unnatural death.

The Coroner is appointed by the local authority, but he can only be dismissed by the Lord Chancellor. He may be either a lawyer or a doctor of not less than five years' standing; the majority of Coroners are solicitors but certain Coroners, notably in London, are doubly qualified, in medicine and law.

Coroner's procedure

The Coroner is empowered to enquire into the cause and circumstances of any death, when the cause is obscure or apparently unnatural, and into the death of a prisoner.

Once the death has been notified to the Coroner, preliminary enquiries are made on his behalf by his officer. This officer is usually a serving police officer, seconded either whole-time, or only during the investigation of a particular case. The scene of death, and the body of the deceased, are viewed, statements taken from witnesses, and a police report is submitted to the Coroner. Usually a post-mortem examination of the deceased is performed by a pathologist, on the instructions of the Coroner.

If the result of the enquiry is to show that death is due to a natural cause, the Coroner will usually conclude the enquiry by issuing his 'Pink form' (Form 100 Part B), which is a certificate of cause of death, for the purpose of registration of the death. He may also issue an order for burial, or, if disposal is to be by cremation, Form E which replaces Forms B and C under the regulations of the Cremation Acts.

The Coroner is entitled to hold an inquest on any case which is reported to him, but in practice usually only does so when the cause of death is unnatural. In certain circumstances, e.g. a road traffic accident, or the death of a prisoner, he is obliged by law to hold an inquest, usually with a jury. Before holding an inquest he must view the body.

Coroner's inquest

In large cities the Coroner has his own courtroom, but elsewhere he may conduct his inquest in any convenient place, other than licensed premises, e.g. a police station, hospital boardroom, Magistrate's Court, etc. The Coroner's Officer keeps order in the Court, marshals the witnesses, and may administer the oath to them.

A witness must take the oath, or affirm, according to his religious conviction. His evidence is given in the form of answers to questions put to him by the Coroner. Lawyers may attend the Court to represent interested parties, and may at the discretion of the Coroner question the witness, and the Coroner may also allow questions to be put by relatives, or the foreman of the jury. The witness must answer all questions put to him, except for those which, if answered, might force him to incriminate himself.

The medical practitioner usually required to give evidence at an inquest is the pathologist who performed the post-mortem examination, but any general practitioner or hospital doctor may find himself summoned to an inquest to give evidence about the death of one of his patients. Such a summons must be obeyed; failure to comply constitutes contempt of court. The doctor should take care to refresh his mind of the facts of the case before giving evidence. His attendance is never required as a mere formality. Also he should take with him all relevant documents which he possesses, e.g. medical records, X-rays, etc.

He must not be misled by the apparent informality of the proceedings, an impression liable to be fostered by the location of the inquest, and the fact that the Coroner and any lawyers present are not robed. He must give careful thought to the statements that he makes, because (a) they are made on oath, and deliberate falsehood is then perjury, and (b) the record of evidence (the deposition) may be relevant in any subsequent criminal or civil proceedings. Ill-considered opinions and statements made in the Coroner's Court may have far-reaching consequences, and may be the starting point of lengthy, costly, and pointless litigation.

After giving evidence, the doctor will usually be released by the Coroner, but may not leave the Court without such permission.

The Coroner's duty at his inquest is restricted to determining who the deceased was, when and where he died, and the cause of death. He has power, when sitting with a jury, to commit a person to the Crown Court on a charge of murder, manslaughter, or infanticide, but cannot consider or decide questions of civil liability. Therefore the possibility that a doctor has been negligent will not be considered in the Coroner's Court, unless the facts indicate criminal negligence. Nevertheless, evidence given in the Court may form the basis for subsequent litigation at a civil court, or for criminal proceedings, and in such circumstances the doctor is entitled and would be well advised to be legally represented at the inquest.

The fees payable to witnesses are fixed by law.

In Scotland a different procedure exists. The Procurator-Fiscal is the official who is responsible for investigating sudden deaths. Should he require a public enquiry or an autopsy, he applies to the Sheriff, who holds the Enquiry, with a jury, and who issues authorisation for the performance of an autopsy.

Magistrate's Court

In these Courts the bulk of the minor criminal work is carried out, and also more serious cases proceeding to the Crown Court for trial are examined to ensure that there really is a *prima facie* (i.e. an apparently genuine) case against the accused. The doctor may be required to give evidence in the Magistrate's Court at such preliminary hearings, or 'committals', and also in cases of alleged drunkenness, assault, sexual offences, etc.

The Court is presided over by one or more magistrates, or justices of the peace, who are not lawyers. They have a Clerk of the Court, a lawyer, to advise them on legal matters. Lawyers, who are usually solicitors, conduct the prosecution and the defence.

The doctor, when called, will take the oath, and will then be questioned first by the prosecuting solicitor. He will then be cross-examined by the defending solicitor, and may also be questioned by the magistrate, who should be addressed as 'Your Worship' or 'Sir'.

If the case in which the doctor is giving evidence is a 'committal', he must remember to speak slowly, as his evidence is being taken down as he speaks, usually on a typewriter, by the Clerk. When his evidence is concluded, this record, known as his deposition, will be read back to him and if it is correct he must sign it. Therefore he must be sure that it is a true record of his statements and opinions, as it will be used as the basis of his evidence at the higher Court, and departure from it there will cause adverse comment.

Crown Courts

As a result of the Courts Act 1971, these replaced the Quarter Sessions and Assize Courts. There are three tiers of Crown Courts, the first tier resembling the old Assize Courts in that the court can try criminal or civil cases, and is presided over by a High Court Judge.

All the more serious criminal cases except treason, e.g. murder, rape, robbery with violence, etc., are dealt with at Crown Courts, and are tried by a jury. Barristers conduct the prosecution and the defence, and are known as counsel.

A doctor may be called to give evidence by either the prosecution or the defence. His evidence will usually have been given earlier in statements to the police and in evidence given in the lower court (the Magistrate's Court) when the case was first heard at the committal stage, and that evidence forms the basis of his examination at the Court.

No matter which side calls him, it is important that the doctor gives his evidence in an impartial and objective manner, stating the facts clearly, and his conclusions drawn from them, without concern as to whether they favour one or other side. If he appears to be biased he will be liable to severe cross-examination, and his opinions will be suspect.

When warned to attend the Court to give evidence (the warning will probably only be given on the evening before the case is to be heard), the doctor would be well-advised to refresh his mind on the facts of the case, especially since the case will probably not come to trial until several months after the alleged crime was committed. For this reason it is also essential that the doctor should have accurate and reliable notes to which he may refer. On arriving at court the following day, the doctor should be prepared for a long wait, since the case may involve ten or twenty witnesses, and may last for two days or even longer.

When called into Court the doctor should take with him into the witness box all the relevant notes, reports and X-rays of the case. He is allowed to refer in the box to reports and X-rays, and to notes made at the time of the examination, to refresh his memory. He will be questioned first by the counsel of the party which has called him. This is known as the examination-in-chief, and during this the relevant medical facts, and the conclusions which the doctor has drawn from these facts are elicited.

Next the counsel for the other party will cross-examine the doctor. He will ask questions designed to test whether any examinations ot tests, which might lead to a different interpretation of the case, have been omitted, and whether any alternative conclusions could be tenable on the facts. Finally the doctor may be re-examined by the first counsel, to clear up points which may have arisen during cross-examination. At any stage the Judge may interpose, to disallow a question for legal reasons, or to clarify a point. He must be addressed as 'My Lord'. If the doctor feels he cannot answer a question without betraying professional secrecy, then he should appeal to the Judge, and must act as he directs.

Barristers are courteous and correct, and provided that the doctor knows his facts, he need not fear their examination. He in his turn must be polite when answering questions, and be prepared to admit any alternative explanation of the facts which is reasonable, when put to him even if he had not thought of it.

He must be careful to speak slowly, so that he may be audible, and also to aid the shorthand writer, who has to make a record of all that is said. Whenever practicable he must also restrict himself to simple words and avoid technical terms and phrases, since the jury will not understand them. For instance it is better to describe an incised wound as a 'cut', or a metacarpo-phalangeal joint as a 'knuckle'.

When the doctor's evidence has been given, the counsel for the party who called the doctor will normally ask the Judge if the doctor may be released, to return to his practice. Whether the doctor does so, or has to remain in the Court, he should refrain from speaking to witnesses who have not yet given evidence, lest collusion be suggested.

Civil Courts

The majority of these are County Courts, and are presided over by County Court Judges, who are addressed as 'Your Honour'. These courts deal with all the relatively minor matters of civil litigation, the more serious cases going to the High Court. The form of the procedure is much the same as in the criminal courts. The advocates may be either solicitors or barristers. The doctor who is called to give evidence will be examined, cross-examined and re-examined in the same way as in the other courts. Questions of compensation and of negligence will come to such courts, and the medical evidence is likely to be more concerned with balance of probabilities than in the criminal courts, where proof is required. There-fore it is likely that each party will obtain the services of a doctor. In such an event it is important to avoid dispute and wrangling. The doctor should ensure that the views he expresses are in accord with the facts and should firmly but politely adhere to his conclusions.

At all times when giving evidence in any court the doctor should remember that his sole purpose is to aid the court in arriving at a just decision, by describing and explaining the medical aspects of the case, and the conclusions which can be drawn from them. Whether these support one or other side in a dispute should be quite immaterial to him.

He should remember that it is no disgrace to have to admit that he does not know the answer to any particular question, and that to admit this at once is infinitely preferable to being forced to admit ignorance after a prolonged attempt to evade the issue. Moreover he should never attempt to answer questions on subjects which are outside his sphere of competence.

CHAPTER 11
Drunkenness

Drunkenness is of medico-legal importance, partly because a drunken person is particularly liable to sustain injuries or to have accidents which may result in death or serious injury, and indeed he may die from the effects of the alcohol alone; and partly because the person may commit various offences while under the influence of alcohol.

Therefore at any time a doctor, whether in general practice or in a hospital department, may be required to examine a person suspected of being drunk. Where possible such an examination is better performed by a doctor accustomed to the procedure, such as a police surgeon, but this may not be possible, and so every doctor should have an elementary knowledge of how to make the examination. Otherwise not only is he liable to appear ridiculous when giving evidence in court, but he is liable to mistake some serious illness for drunkenness, with the result that the person will not receive appropriate treatment and may die.

Persons who are drunk may sustain serious injury or die because of:

1   Head injuries—e.g. extra or sub-dural haemorrhage following falls or fights. Not only will the drunken person be more aggressive or unsteady, but the presence of alcohol in the body makes bleeding more likely to occur, and in a chronic alcoholic the blood vessels may have become more fragile.

2   Falls from buildings, into areas or excavations, etc., may produce fractures, especially of the skull or neck.

3   Drowning—the drunken person may blunder into a river or canal. He may also collapse insensible in the street with his face in a puddle or gutter, and drown in a few inches of water.

4   Burns—by falls into fires or dropping cigarettes or lighted matches.

5   Electrocution—by fumbling with faulty apparatus.

6   Poisoning—commonly from carbon monoxide, by switching on the gas but forgetting to light it. Also by drinking other poisons in mistake for water or further supplies of alcohol.

7   Asphyxia—from becoming trapped in confined spaces, becoming accidentally suspended, e.g. by clothing, smothering from bedclothes, strangulation from tight clothing during the alcoholic coma, or choking from the regurgitation and inhalation of stomach contents.

Drunkenness and the law

To be drunk is not an offence, unless the drunken person is behaving or performing some action to the annoyance or danger of other persons.

Drunken driving

Under the provisions of the Road Traffic Act 1972 it is an offence for a person to drive or attempt to drive a motor vehicle on a road or other public place if he is unfit to drive through drink or drugs; it is also an offence if he has an amount of alcohol in his blood greater than the prescribed limit, which is 80 mg of alcohol in 100 ml of blood (equivalent to 107 mg of alcohol in 100 ml of urine).

A police constable who suspects a motorist of having alcohol in his body or having committed a traffic offence can require him to take a breath test. If the breath test is positive the constable can arrest the motorist, and, at the police station require him to supply a blood or urine sample, for analysis. Refusal to supply any of the samples is an offence, but if the motorist has been admitted to hospital the police constable must obtain the permission of the medical officer in charge of the patient before requesting any of the samples, and the medical officer can refuse permission if this would be prejudicial to the treatment of the patient.

The role of a doctor in this procedure is restricted to obtaining a blood sample with consent from the patient, and this responsibility usually devolves on the police surgeon. At the time when the sample is taken, in addition to the specimen handed to the police, part of the sample must be given to the motorist, in a sealed container, to enable him to obtain an independent analysis.

Drunk in various situations

Drunkenness may constitute an offence if on a passenger steamer, or in control of a child under 7 years, or in possession of loaded firearms, or in charge of horse or cattle, etc.

Overlaying of children

Under the Children and Young Persons Act any adult, over the age of 16, who, while under the influence of alcohol, takes a child under the age of 3 years into bed, as a result of which the child is suffocated by being overlayed, commits an offence.

In crimes of violence—e.g. murder

Normally the fact that a person's mental attitude may be modified by alcohol, e.g. he may become more aggressive and so attack another, is not considered to reduce his responsibility for his actions. However it may be proved that at the time of the occurrence the accused was so hopelessly drunk as to be quite incapable of knowing what he was doing, or of forming any specific intention. This may reduce the offence from murder to manslaughter. Chronic alcoholism may amount to true insanity.

The physiology of alcohol

Alcohol is usually rapidly absorbed from the stomach, though this absorption may be slowed down if the stomach contains a meal, or especially fat, such as milk or olive oil. Most of a dose of alcohol will be absorbed from the stomach in 1 hour.

The alcohol then becomes distributed throughout the body, in proportion to the amount of water present in various tissues.

Elimination of the alcohol from the body is slower than its absorption. Most is metabolised, the average rate being 10 ml per hour, equal to a fall of 15 mg per 100 ml per hour in the blood level of alcohol. There is considerable individual variation, however. About 90% of the ingested alcohol is removed in this way, the rest is excreted in the urine, breath and sweat.

Ratio between blood and urine alcohol levels (figure 3)

During the time that alcohol is being absorbed the amount in the blood exceeds that in the urine. But once absorption ceases and elimination commences the level in the urine becomes greater than that in the blood at a given time in the ratio 4 : 3, since the urine obtained at a particular time is derived from blood passing through the kidneys some appreciable time before, when the blood level was higher. This is likely to apply at the time when the doctor makes his examination, and the known ratio makes it possible to calculate the level in the blood from an examination of the urine only. However, if there is any possibility of doubt then it is as well to take blood as well as urine samples.

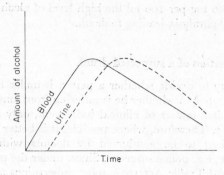

FIG. 3

Relation of blood alcohol level to symptoms

This will depend to a large extent on the person under examination, and how accustomed he is to taking alcohol, whether he is tired, or cold, or has taken any other drugs at the same time, or has disease such as cerebral-arterio-sclerosis.

0–50 mg per 100 ml of blood—no symptoms likely

50–150 mg per 100 ml of blood—the levels usually reached during normal social drinking. The alcohol has produced some depression of higher centres and the person is talkative, and aggressive or friendly. The face and eyes are slightly suffused and there is a tendency to nystagmus, with dilated pupils.

150–250 mg per 100 ml of blood—at this stage the person is intoxicated, as shown by muscular incoordination, slurred speech, impairment of memory, etc.

250–400 mg per 100 ml of blood—the person at this level has reached the stage of pre-coma, is grossly incoordinated with incoherent speech and sluggishly reacting pupils.

400–500 mg per 100 ml of blood—the stage of coma has now been reached, with slow stertorous breathing, pallor, subnormal temperature and contracted pupils.

Over 500 mg per 100 ml the high level of alcohol causes medullary paralysis, leading to death.

Examination of a suspected drunk

The ability to decide whether a person is under the influence of alcohol, or whether he is suffering from some disease or injury is a matter of clinical judgement, only acquired by practice. Therefore, where possible, it is better for such examinations to be conducted by doctors with special experience, e.g. police surgeons. Since, under the provisions of the Road Traffic Act 1972, most prosecutions are likely to be based on the results of analysis of blood or urine samples, clinical examinations to assess drunkenness are much less frequently required than formerly. However, in special circumstances a doctor may be required to make such an examination. The following notes only give the very general outline of the procedure. For greater detail the student should consult the B.M.A. pamphlet, *The Recognition of Intoxication* (1954).

Time

If requested to make the examination the doctor should attend as quickly as possible, since the effects of intoxication may begin to wear off, and if the patient is suffering from some other condition he may be in danger. The time when the doctor is called, and when he begins his examination should be recorded.

Consent

Before making any examination the doctor should obtain the consent of the patient, in writing and witnessed. He must explain the nature and the purpose of the examination he proposes to make and that his findings will be made known to the police. He must also explain what samples he proposes to take.

The doctor must at this stage make it clear that the patient is not obliged to submit to an examination, and that he is entitled to insist that the examination is conducted by a doctor of his own choice.

If the patient is incapable of giving consent by reason of unconsciousness or gross intoxication, then the doctor may make an examination, take samples, and give such treatment as is necessary to save life. However, he may not divulge the results of his examination until he can obtain the consent of the patient, or the patient dies, except when directed to do so by a court.

Purpose of the examination

The aim of the doctor should be to decide whether the patient is under the influence of alcohol, and if so to what extent, e.g. is his ability to drive properly impaired; or is his condition due to illness or injury; and is it safe for him to be detained in a police station, or should he be admitted to hospital.

Form of the examination

(as given in the B.M.A. pamphlet)

1   The presence of any serious injury or acute illness requiring immediate attention should be excluded at once.
2   History, e.g. of previous illnesses, fits, etc., of the nature of any recent food or drink, and whether the patient is taking any drugs.
3   General behaviour—state of dress, speech and self-control.
4   Memory and mental state—questions of name and address, date and time, and simple arithmetic.
5   Writing—copying from book or newspaper.
6   Pulse—temperature—skin condition.

D

7 Mouth—state of tongue, nature of teeth, smell of breath.

8 Eyes—general appearance, glass eyes, pupil reactions, eye movements.

9 Ears—impairment of hearing, condition of drums.

10 Gait—on walking across a room and turning (not along a straight line).

11 Stance—with eyes open and closed.

12 Co-ordination—finger-nose test, picking up objects, performing simple acts such as buttoning clothing.

13 Reflexes—and general CNS examination.

14 Examinations of cardiovascular, respiratory and alimentary systems.

Diagnosis

This must be based on the whole of the results of the examination, not on isolated features such as the smell of the breath.

The doctor's report to the police must only deal with matters for which he was asked to make the examination, e.g. the presence of intoxication, the presence of other disease, and the fitness of the person to be detained. These opinions must only relate to the patient at the time of the examination. No opinion should be given of the patient's condition at some time earlier than the examination.

Specimens

These usually consist of urine or breath samples, and arrangements for obtaining these will have been made by the police, so that the doctor is not concerned. Blood samples may be requested by the police or by the patient, and can only be taken with the consent of the patient. The sample must be divided into two, one part being given to the police, the other to the patient. The object is to allow the person to obtain an independent analysis if he wishes.

Alcohol must not be used to sterilise the skin or the syringe, of course.

The patient may refuse to allow a sample to be taken, but this may be taken by the court subsequently to support the prosecution's case, or may constitute an offence under the provisions of the Road Traffic Act 1972.

'Special' kits containing receptacles for the blood, etc., are held by the police. The receptacles must contain flouride to prevent enzymatic decomposition of the blood. After filling they must be kept cool, but not frozen or heated. Once in the sealed container, the seal must not be broken until the sample reaches the analyst.

CHAPTER 12
Sexual Offences

Types of offence

These are set out in the Sexual Offences Act, 1956, as amended by the Sexual Offences Act, 1967, in respect of homosexual acts.

Rape

This has been defined as unlawful sexual intercourse with a woman by force and against her will. It is a crime which carries a maximum punishment of life imprisonment.

Note that:

1 Sexual intercourse, within the meaning of the Act, is constituted by any degree of penetration from mere entry of the tip of the penis between the labia majora to full

penetration into the vagina, with or without emission of seminal fluid. The point is that conception may occur without full penetration, if semen is deposited at the vulva, and moreover, the degree of emotional shock may be equally great whether or not full penetration has occurred.

2   Sexual intercourse with an adult woman may be lawful, if she gives consent, and is always lawful in marriage unless the parties are legally separated, the marriage contract implying consent of the wife to intercourse. Therefore a man cannot rape his wife, though his conduct may constitute cruelty, sufficient to justify divorce, or the offences of wounding or assault, or causing grievous bodily harm.

3   'By force and against her will' includes not only the actual use of bodily violence to restrain or coerce the woman, but also the threat of violence, and also includes the use of drugs to stupefy the woman, and the use of fraud such as impersonation of the husband.

Intercourse with children

Intercourse with girls under the age of 16 years is always illegal, even if consent is given; such consent is always invalid. However, girls who are close to 16 years of age may dress and behave as though they were much older, and deceive the unwary male. Therefore the law creates two classes of offence.

(a) Intercourse with a girl under 13 years of age. This is considered a grave offence, ranking with rape.

(b) Intercourse with a girl between 13 and 16 years of age, unless accomplished by force and against her will, in which case it will be rape, is a less grave offence, punishable with up to 2 years' imprisonment.

There may be a valid defence to a charge of this latter offence, if it is shown that the accused man was under 24 years, he genuinely believed and had reasonable cause to believe that the girl was over 16 years old, and he had never before been *charged* with a like offence.

Intercourse with mental defectives

It is an offence, punishable by 2 years' imprisonment, for a man to have intercourse with a woman who is suffering from mental subnormality or severe subnormality, or a patient under the care of a mental hospital, or under guardianship unless it can be shown that the man was not aware of the mental state of the woman.

Incest

It is an offence for a man to have intercourse with his granddaughter, daughter, sister, half-sister or mother.

Similarly a woman may not have intercourse with her grandson, son, brother, half-brother or father.

If intercourse is with a girl under 13 years of age, then as before, this is a grave offence punishable by life imprisonment, otherwise punishment may be up to 7 years' imprisonment.

Indecent assault

This offence can be committed by either a man or a woman. Indeed a woman cannot be charge with the rape of a man or boy, but can be charged with indecent assault.

The range of acts constituting such an assault is wide, from handling the genitalia to merely disarranging the clothing.

As in the case of sexual intercourse, an adult woman can give consent to such behaviour, as in courtship, and in that case no offence is committed. However, girls under the age of 16 years, and mental defectives, cannot give valid consent for such behaviour, which in their case, therefore, always constitutes an offence.

Because the range of acts constituting such an offence is so wide, any persons who have to examine or interview members of the opposite sex, such as doctors, are always at risk from false or mistaken allegations of misconduct, unless the utmost care is taken with regard to chaperons, etc. Doctors and dentists are particularly as risk when administering anaesthetics to female patients, since erotic dreams, followed by discovery of disordered clothing on recovering consciousness, may lead to the genuinely mistaken belief on the patient's part that she has been assaulted.

Examination of an alleged victim of sexual offence

Before conducting such an examination, remember:

1   Many allegations of rape are false, possibly as many as 11 out of 12. Such allegations may be from spite, jealousy, in order to precipitate marriage, etc.

2   The doctor must endeavour to show whether or not sexual intercourse has taken place, and to note any injuries. He cannot say whether rape has occurred. Penetration and emission of semen with bruises and teeth marks may occur in consenting intercourse. Equally, a rape can occur without full penetration or emission and without the production of any injuries.

3   The offence charged is a grave one, therefore if possible these examinations should only be performed by doctors having special experience of such cases.

The scheme of examination

Consent. Obtain written consent from the girl, or her parent or guardian if she is under 16 years.

Premises. Ensure that the examination can be conducted in suitable premises, such as the doctor's surgery; not in some ill-lit waiting-room of a police station.

History. Take a history of the occurrence, if possible, both from the girl and separately from some other person in whom she has confided, e.g. the mother. Note both the date and time of the examination, and also the date and time of the alleged incident.

It is important to know, for instance:

(a) The place of the incident; house, wood, etc.
(b) The course of events during the incident.
(c) The relative position of the parties.
(d) The steps taken by the victim to resist.
(e) Whether the victim lost consciousness at any time.
(f) Whether she was menstruating at the time.

General Appearance. While taking the history, note the general appearance and behaviour of the girl, signs of distress or discomfort, apparent age and physique, and whether she dresses or looks older than her age.

Clothing. Enquire whether the clothing worn at the examination is that worn when the attack occurred. If so, it should be examined for damage, tears, stains, etc., and arrangements made for it to be sent to a Forensic Science Laboratory for examination, ensuring that it is safely packed to avoid contamination, in polythene bags, and labelled, with the doctor's initials or identifying mark on the label to allow identification subsequently in court.

Physical Examination. (i) General. It is important to examine the whole of the body for injuries, notably bruises and abrasions, especially on the thighs, from separating the legs, on the arms from gripping, on the back of the shoulders from forcibly holding down, and on the face and neck from prevention of the woman crying out. Also bite or suction marks, oval bruises, may be found on the neck or on the breasts, and the nipples may be bitten. Note her physique, in relation to the amount of resistance of which she would be capable.

(ii) Of the genitalia. This follows the pattern of a normal gynaecological examination, but especially noting:

(a) Pubic hair. Any matting by semen. Remember to take

a sample, but not until the end of the examination, since the hairs should be plucked, not cut.

(b) Vulva. Look for swelling, reddening, abrasions, lacerations, and tenderness.

(c) Hymen. Look for a fresh tear of the hymen, with reddening and tenderness of the margins. Old tears are of no assistance, and in a married woman the hymen may be absent. Even if a virgin it may be so elastic or small as to be undamaged by intercourse.

(d) Vagina. Look for bruising, abrasion, or laceration of the walls. Dilatation of the vagina is not necessarily proof of intercourse, it may be due to the use of tampons or masturbation. A sample of vaginal fluid should be taken for examination for spermatozoa. The sample may be taken either by capillary pipette, and smears prepared on microscope slides, or by means of a damp throat swab. In either case, if the sample has to be sent any distance to the laboratory, smears should be prepared at once, and allowed to dry on the slides, otherwise the sperms will disintegrate.

The swabs should be sent as well as the smears, however, so that bacteriological examination can be made for venereal disease, and if this is thought possible it would be as well for the swabs to be sent in some transport medium.

Any fibres or foreign hairs found on the genitalia should be preserved and sent for examination, as well as a sample of the girl's pubic hair, and also a blood sample for grouping.

Remember. The object of the examination is (a) to determine whether intercourse has taken place, by finding seminal fluid in the vagina, (b) to note any injuries to the body or genitalia denoting forceful intercourse, or a struggle, but remembering that such injuries do not necessarily indicate rape.

Examination of a person accused of rape

It is unlikely a doctor will be called upon to make such an examination unless he is a police surgeon or prison medical officer. However, the general principles of such an examination are as follows:

(a) *Obtain written consent* for the examination, after explaining its purpose.

(b) If possible, take a history of the circumstances of the intercourse. The man's story may accord better with the facts than the girl's.

(c) Note any stains on the clothing. Their identification is a job for the Forensic Science Laboratory.

(d) Note the man's age and physique. Look for injuries which might have been sustained during a struggle, such as nail scratches on the face.

(e) Note the size of the penis, and whether or not the man is potent. Examine for injuries to the penis, such as a tear of the frenum. Look for evidence of active venereal disease.

(f) Take samples of pubic hair, and also blood samples for grouping.

Anal intercourse

Sexual intercourse per anum has always been regarded as unnatural, and a crime of considerable gravity, a felony known as buggery. It was immaterial whether the act was performed on a man or a woman. However, the Sexual Offences Act 1967, recognising the existence and needs of homosexual persons, has made the act lawful as between consenting adults, performed in private. (A public lavatory is specifically excluded as a private place.)

It is still unlawful for the act to be performed on a person who does not give consent, including those, i.e. children, who cannot give consent. The age at which a person becomes an adult for the purposes of this Act is 21 years. (A boy under 14 is sexually immature and cannot be accused of rape, or of buggery. He can be accused of indecent assault.)

Therefore, the doctor may be called upon to examine a person who alleges anal intercourse has been practised on him without his consent, and also possibly the person who is alleged to have performed the act.

Medical examination

The passive agent. If seen soon after an act of anal intercourse, performed for the first time, the anal wall may be painful, reddened, grazed and bruised. There may be small fresh tears of the wall. There may be traces of lubricant in the anal canal, such as petroleum jelly, and also seminal fluid, which must be retained for examination on slides or a swab as in the case of rape.

Where anal intercourse is frequently practised, the anal canal becomes dilated and its walls scarred, due to old tears. It will tend to dilate when the buttocks are separated. There may be evidence of venereal disease. The doctor must beware mistaking natural disease, such as anal fissure or rectal prolapse, for evidence of anal intercourse.

The active agent. Little is likely to be found here, except possibly fresh injury to the penis and traces of faecal material on the glans.

Bestiality

This is sexual intercourse with animals, a form of sexual perversion obviously more likely to be encountered in the country. Proof is usually a matter of investigation by the police and by Forensic Scientists, and the doctor is not likely to be involved.

PART TWO
Forensic Pathology

CHAPTER 13
Examination of the Dead

The first and principal duty of a doctor who is called to the scene of a death is to ascertain that death has in fact occurred. Lack of care in this examination has caused some embarrassing moments when 'bodies' have revived in the mortuary, notably of persons suffering from hypothermia, electrocution or poisoning. If the person is still alive, or the fact of death is not certain after examination, the doctor's only concern should be the welfare of the patient.

Two types of death are described, somatic death which is extinction of personality when vital processes cease, and molecular death, when the tissues of the body begin to disintegrate. The diagnosis of somatic death is of greater practical importance, and with modern apparatus for transfusion, artificial respiration, cardiac stimulation, etc., it may be difficult to decide at what moment a person has ceased to be an individual, and has become a mass of tissues being artificially maintained by the therapeutic procedures.

Signs of death

Death is considered to have occurred when the vital functions, e.g. breathing and heart-beat, have irreversibly ceased. In hospital this may if necessary be firmly established by the use of investigations such as E.C.G. or E.E.G. Otherwise the absence of any heart or breath sounds on auscultation over a period of five minutes is sufficient indication. Other old-fashioned tests such as mirrors or feathers on the mouth or ligatures around the finger are quite unreliable.

Examination of the eye with an ophthalmoscope may

confirm the cessation of the circulation by showing breaking up of the columns of blood in the retinal blood vessels.

If there is any doubt, e.g. dubious heart sounds heard during an examination in a noisy street, it is obviously safer to assume that the person is still alive and send him at once to hospital where E.E.G. or even auscultation in quiet surroundings may settle the issue.

Associated with the failure of vital functions are the pallor of the skin, flaccidity of muscles and dilated pupils which make up the 'dead' appearance, but which are too imprecise to serve as criteria for the diagnosis of death.

Bodily changes after death

Some of the earlier of these changes, such as cooling of the body, and rigor mortis, are confirmatory evidence that death has occurred. All of them are of value in indicating approximately when death occurred.

Cooling

Theoretically this starts as soon as life ceases, and continues for about 18–24 hours, until the body temperature reaches that of its surroundings, at an average rate of $1\cdot5°F$ per hour. The actual rate may vary between about $3°F$ and $\frac{1}{2}°F$ per hour, depending on whether death has only recently occurred, or took place many hours previously, i.e. the difference in temperature between the body and its surroundings is great or little. The rate of fall will also be slowed in a well-clothed body or one which is fat, and hastened in a naked or thin body, or one immersed in water.

To obtain a rough approximation of the time of death, from the extent of cooling, divide the number of degrees of temperature lost from $99°F$ by $1\cdot5$ (i.e. allowing for a rate of cooling of $1\cdot5°F$ per hour). But it must be remembered that this is only an approximation; the body may not commence to cool for several hours after death, or the tempera-

ture at or soon after death may exceed the normal 98·4°F
by up to 7°F. Therefore these factors can introduce an
error of several hours in the estimated time of death. The
temperature must be recorded in the rectum, not on the
body surface, using a long chemical thermometer, or a low-
reading variety.

Hypostasis

After death blood drains in the relaxed and dilated vessels
by gravity to the lowest parts of the body. This process
starts at death, but is not normally apparent for 4–6 hours,
and is fully established in about 12 hours. After 12 hours the
blood becomes coagulated in the vessels, so that if a body is
rolled over after this time the hypostasis will not alter its
distribution, and will be seen on the uppermost part of the
body. The hypostasis is often difficult to see in a fat person
or one who has lost much blood recently. Its colour may
indicate chemical changes in the blood during life, e.g. pink
due to carboxyhaemoglobin or grey-brown due to methaemoglobin.

Rigor Mortis

This stiffening of the muscles is due to coagulation of muscle
protein by substances derived from breakdown of glucose,
notably lactic acid. It affects the smaller muscles of the jaw
and the extremities before the larger muscle masses. Under
normal conditions the stiffening will be apparent in about 6
hours, and will have affected the whole body in 12 hours.
This stiffness of the body will last for about 36–48 hours,
before passing off as putrefaction begins to dissolve the
muscle protein. This time-pattern is however subject to
considerable variation. A person who has been using his
muscles violently, e.g. in fight or flight, will have an accumulation of the products of glucose metabolism already
present in the muscles at death, and so rigor will develop

more rapidly. For the same reasons certain poisons such as strychnine will hasten the onset of rigor. On the other hand slow lingering deaths, where the muscle supplies of glucose are depleted, will be associated with slower and weaker development of rigor. Also the rate at which rigor passes off will obviously be related to the speed of onset of putrefaction, which may be very rapid in hot environments.

Once a stiffened muscle, in rigor, is stretched, and the rigor 'broken' stiffening will not recur.

Other causes of stiffening of muscles:

1 In extensive burns, where the heat 'cooks' the muscle protein.

2 In intense cold when the joints are frozen; on thawing the muscles will pass into rigor.

3 Cadaveric spasm; a rare condition of unknown mechanism, in which in sudden violent deaths, groups of muscles or the whole body may suddenly stiffen at the moment of death, e.g. the hand holding a weapon used in a suicidal attempt.

Putrefaction

The presence of this process is not likely to be in doubt, when fully developed. Its early stages consist of a greenish discoloration of the skin of the anterior abdominal wall over the right iliac fossa, soon spreading to the whole of the abdominal wall, appearing at about 48 hours after death in normal conditions. Subsequently the body swells and discoloration appears along the lines of the superficial veins (marbling), with blistering of the skin, rupture of body cavities and liquefaction of organs.

The temperature of the environment will of course affect the speed of onset of the putrefaction.

Adipocere

This change does not occur for several weeks or months

after death. It consists of a hydrolysis of body fats to fatty acids and soaps, the end product, adipocere, being a white greasy musty-smelling material, which by replacing the fatty tissue, may maintain the outline of the part or even the whole of the body. It is most commonly found in bodies lying in relatively warm moist anaerobic situations, e.g. clothed bodies buried in poorly drained soil. If the soil is very acid, e.g. peat bog, an alternative process akin to tanning may preserve the entire body in an excellent state, as in certain archaeological discoveries in Denmark.

In warm, dry environments, the body may become dry and brittle, and dark brown in colour, the process being known as mummification.

Post-mortem mutilation

After death a body may be exposed to the attacks of animals and insects. The animals, either domestic, such as cats, or wild as rats or foxes, may cause severe damage, during the first few days after death, which can be distinguished from injuries caused in life by the presence of minute scratches or toothmarks at the margins of the injuries. The onset of putrefaction may be accompanied by infestation by maggots or beetle larvae.

Estimating the time of death—survey

Death	
0–12 hr	Body temperature
24 hr	Rigor mortis and hypostasis
48 hr–3 wk	Putrefaction
months–years	Adipocere and mummification

Visiting the scene of death

This is likely to occur in one of two circumstances:

1 On a routine visit to see the body of a dead patient before the doctor issues a death certificate, where there are no suspicious circumstances.

2 Visiting the scene of a death in suspicious circumstances, summoned by the police.

Circumstances not suspicious

Obviously such cases are almost always ordinary deaths from natural causes, and to treat each one in a manner that implied to the relatives that one suspected foul play would be ridiculous. However unless the doctor was actually present at the moment of death, he should always have suspicions, though keeping them to himself. Thus having confirmed the fact of death he should check the body to eliminate the presence of any injuries, examining especially the neck, and the back of the body. He should note any tablets or cups in the room or by the bed, which might indicate that poison had been taken, and should see if the deceased had left any notes. He should be especially careful in deaths in young women, since an attempted abortion may leave very little external evidence. (See Chapter 21.) He should not omit to ask any relatives or neighbours for details of the death, and if he is in any doubt about the cause of death, he should inform the Coroner. Common causes of sudden unexpected death are myocardial ischaemia due to coronary atheroma or coronary thrombosis, pulmonary embolism due to leg vein thrombosis, cerebral haemorrhage due to aneurysm or hypertension, and ruptured abdominal aneurysms. Severe infections such as pneumonia or peritonitis may develop rapidly and be unsuspected, especially in elderly persons living on their own. However, the likelihood of a natural cause for sudden death must not blind the doctor to the presence of carbon monoxide poisoning, or a fractured femur.

Suspicious circumstances

In such circumstances the doctor will usually be asked to attend by the police, who are probably treating the case as one of murder until it has been confirmed, or proved otherwise. The principal things for the doctor to bear in mind are:

1 To enquire what is required of him, i.e. is he simply required to establish the fact of death, or to make a more detailed examination.

2 To be sure not to go beyond the scope of his competency, i.e. not to be afraid to admit if he is unfamiliar with the particular type of death.

3 To be careful not to interfere with the investigations of others, i.e. by destroying fingerprints, stains, suicide notes, etc.

It is obviously important to attend at the scene of death as quickly as possible. On arrival the doctor should obtain a brief statement of the circumstances, and enquire what is required of him. He should also enquire what he must not touch, the golden rule being to touch as little as possible and to displace nothing.

His most important function is to ascertain that death has occurred, with as little disturbance as possible. However, if he thinks that life is still present, or he cannot be sure, then all other things must be subordinated to the treatment of the person. If death has undoubtedly occurred, he should try to form an opinion as to the approximate time of death from the state of rigor, body temperature, etc. He should check that the identity of the deceased is correct, and he should endeavour to ascertain the cause of death, from the presence of obvious marks or injuries such as the mark of a ligature on the neck. He should note the position and state of clothing of the body before it is moved, and make a quick sketch plan to refresh his memory later and he should make a note of such things as the type and distribution of any bloodstains, cups, tablets, weapons, etc., in the area.

These things should be recorded in writing as soon as possible, preferably at the scene, with the time of the investigation, the names of the relevant police officers, the address of the premises, etc., so that if the case comes to court in 2 to 3 months' time the doctor can refresh his memory, from his original notes.

Medico-legal autopsy

It is very unlikely that a general practitioner would be called upon to perform a medico-legal autopsy, therefore it is not proposed to make any detailed description of the methods employed. Such an examination should only be performed by a pathologist having special experience in this field. Details of who may be called upon to perform such autopsies, and of the type of examination required are contained in the Coroners Rules (1953). The principles of the examination are:

1   To make precise records of when and where the autopsy was performed, and in whose presence.

2   To remember to examine the clothing.

3   To make a detailed and meticulous external examination of the body, noting especially any marks on the neck, the hands, and the genitalia, and remembering to examine the back of the body and the scalp.

4   To enquire at this stage whether any samples are required by the police, such as specimens of hair or/and nail scrapings, and to give the police opportunity to take photographs, fingerprints, etc.

5   During the internal examination to remember to open all the body cavities, including the skull, to measure the amounts of blood or other fluids present in the cavities, to trace the direction and depth of injuries before the organs are removed, and to measure and record all injuries found however trivial they may appear.

6   To remember to retain the gastric contents and samples of blood and urine while this is possible.

7 To ensure that all the samples are kept separately in clean glass containers, are labelled in a way that will enable the doctor to identify them months later, and are handed to the appropriate police officer, whose name the doctor will record.

8 To retain tissues or organs which have a bearing on the death, e.g. any wounds, or neck structures in cases of strangulation, preserved in a way that will make them of use to any other doctor requiring to see them, e.g. a pathologist acting on behalf of the defence.

Autopsy Report

The report on a medico-legal autopsy follows the same general pattern as any autopsy report, e.g. details of the deceased, external findings, internal findings arranged by systems, and conclusions as to cause of death. The precise form varies from one pathologist to another.

However in medico-legal cases it is important to remember the following:

1 The report is the property of the Coroner, and copies may not be given to anyone else without his permission.

2 So far as is possible, consistent with accuracy, the report should be in simple language, avoiding technical terms, since it will have to be read and understood by various laymen at different stages of the investigation.

CHAPTER 14
Blood

Bloodstains

At the scene of a death the doctor's main duty is to examine the body. Other experts, forensic scientists, fingerprint specialists, police photographers, etc., will be responsible for examining the surroundings, and the doctor must be very careful to avoid inadvertently destroying valuable evidence by handling or moving objects.

However, the interpretation of the nature and distribution of bloodstains, in an attempt to determine the circumstances of the death, may be expected of the doctor, either at the scene, or later, in court.

The different kinds of bloodstains which may be present can be considered under three headings:

1 Blood on and around the body.
2 Blood spots and splashes on walls, furniture, etc.
3 Smears, or trails of blood on floors.

Blood on and around the body

Almost any dead body bearing wounds is likely to be lying in a pool of blood, part of which has probably drained out after death. The absence of such a pool is more noteworthy as it suggests that the body has been moved after death. The amount of blood present in relation to the size of the injury is deceptive; a minor injury such as a ruptured varicose vein or a laceration of an eyebrow may produce a large pool of blood, compared to a much more deeply penetrating stab-wound which may have pierced the aorta but where most of the bleeding is into the body cavities.

It may be useful to note the position of bloodstains on the

body, particularly the linear stains produced by blood running across the body from the wound. For instance, signs of blood having trickled down the legs of a body which is found lying on the floor, with a stab-wound in the chest, indicates that the deceased was upright when the wound was inflicted.

Blood spots and splashes on walls, furniture, etc.

These spots may have been produced by blood dripping from a wounded person who was staggering around the room, from spurts of blood escaping from a severed artery, or as spray from a bloodstained weapon wielded by an assailant. This may be determined from the position and shape of the spots; a line of blood spots on the ceiling are likely to have come from a bloodstained weapon; rounded spots on the floor or flat surfaces of furniture probably were produced by blood dripping from the victim.

The direction in which the blood was travelling, and hence the likely point from which it originated, can be determined from the shape of the blood spots. Thus blood dropping vertically on to a flat surface makes a rounded

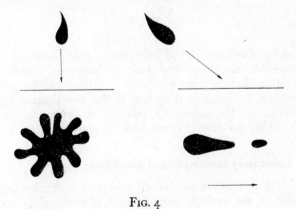

FIG. 4

spot which may have crenated margin if the spot has travelled for some distance. A drop arriving obliquely at the surface will produce a splash in the shape of an exclamation mark !, the smaller spot pointing the direction in which the blood was travelling (figure 4).

Smears and trails of blood on floors

These are produced when the person crawls, or his body is dragged, after wounding. They may consist of a series of drops of blood, or of blood smears on the floor, doorposts, etc. The smears will tend to become indistinct and have a ragged margin in the direction of travel (figure 5).

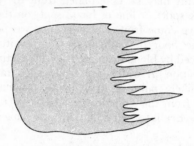

FIG. 5

Apart from noting and interpreting the position of such bloodstains the doctor may have an important function in ensuring that they are preserved until they can be photographed, by pointing them out to the investigating police officers, or by preventing relatives or bystanders from disturbing the scene of death until the police arrive.

Laboratory examination of bloodstains

This is obviously a specialist's field, and a detailed knowledge of the various methods used is never likely to be required by the average doctor. Therefore the following account is only a brief outline of the procedure, designed to indicate the scope of the investigations, and the purpose of preserving samples.

Summary

See figure 6.

Preparation of solution. Before most of the tests can be applied the stain must be taken into solution, by soaking the stained fabric, or fragments of the dried stain scraped from the surface of a weapon or piece of furniture, in normal saline.

Presumptive tests. There are several of these, designed to distinguish stains made by blood or other body fluids from those made by paint, rust, fruit juice, etc.

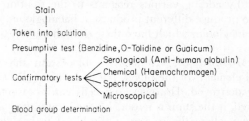

```
                Stain
                  |
        Taken into solution
                  |
Presumptive test (Benzidine,O-Tolidine or Guaicum)
                  |               Serological (Anti-human globulin)
                  |              ╱ Chemical (Haemochromogen)
        Confirmatory tests ⟨
                  |              ╲ Spectroscopical
                  |               Microscopical
        Blood group determination
```

FIG. 6

The best known is the benzidine test. A solution, comprising a mixture of hydrogen peroxide and benzidine dissolved in acetic acid, will give a blue colour with very small quantities of blood. However benzidine is a carcinogenetic substance, the manufacture of which has largely ceased in this country, and a solution of O-tolidine, or guaicum prepared in the same way may be used in its place.

These tests are useful as screening procedures, to

determine which stains deserve further investigation, and also to detect minute traces of blood at a scene, in a wash-basin for instance. A filter-paper may be rubbed on the stain, and the test then applied to the filter-paper.

Confirmatory Tests. (a) *Serological*—These methods are the most commonly used of the various confirmatory procedures, having the merits of speed and specificity. Precipitin tests with anti-human globulin, or other antisera, will confirm that the substance causing the stain is blood, and will indicate whether the blood is human, or animal.

(b) *Chemical*—There are several different tests. Reagents are used to produce derivatives of haemoglobin which have characteristic crystalline forms, visible by microscopic examination. A well-known example of such a method is Takayama's haemochromogen test.

(c) *Spectroscopic*—A solution of reduced haemoglobin has a characteristic absorption spectrum. The test is made more specific by adding various reagents to the solution of the stain, to produce different products of haemoglobin, such as methaemoglobin, which have their own characteristic spectrum.

(d) *Microscopical*—In a dried bloodstain the various formed elements of the blood, red and white cells, etc., are usually destroyed. However, red cells can occasionally be identified, if the stain is reasonably fresh, and their appearance may allow the source of the blood to be identified. Thus the red cells of avian blood are nucleated, and those from a camel are oval (information which is fascinating, but rarely of practical value).

Grouping of bloodstains. Various techniques have been developed by forensic scientists, which depend basically on the absorption by the stain of the specific antibodies from test solutions. The absorbed antibodies are then eluted from the stain, and their presence indicated by agglutination of fresh red cells of known groups.

Thus a dried stain of group B blood will absorb anti-B agglutinins, but not anti-A. The absorbed agglutinins can then be eluted, and will agglutinate known group B red cells.

Such tests can be performed on solutions of the stains, or even on a few fibres from the stained fabric.

The extent of blood-group determination is usually restricted to the ABO system, by the condition of the stains and the amount of material available.

It should be remembered that other body fluids, such as saliva or semen, may contain blood-group substances, and can be grouped in the same way.

Blood samples

From living persons

Such samples are usually required from persons accused of drunken driving, or persons accused of assault or murder. It is important for the doctor who is asked to take such samples to remember:

1 To ensure that the person from whom the sample is to be taken understands the nature of the procedure, and the purpose for which the sample is required, and gives valid consent, in writing.

2 Not to sterilise the skin with alcohol if the sample is later to be analysed for alcohol.

3 To ensure in the case of a 'drunken driver' that the sample is divided into two parts, one to be handed to the police for analysis and one to be given to the accused person so that he may have an independent analysis performed if he wishes.

4 To see that the samples are securely labelled, in a manner that will enable the doctor to identify them later in Court.

5 To make a note of whom he hands the labelled samples to, e.g. the name of the police officer, in case the doctor is asked this in Court, when continuity of evidence is being established.

At Autopsy

Such samples are required either for determination of the deceased's blood group, to compare with the groups of bloodstains on weapons or clothing, or for analysis for alcohol or poisons.

The principles for taking blood samples in the living as regards labelling also apply here. In addition the site from which the blood sample is taken may be important. For grouping purposes it is not necessary that the blood come from any particular site, i.e. it can be taken from the heart or from a peripheral vein, but when taking samples for alcohol estimation the blood should only be taken from a peripheral vein, if possible the femoral vein, to avoid the confusion which may arise from the post-mortem changes in alcohol content, which may occur in the blood in the vicinity of the liver. If other poisons are suspected samples of blood from the heart and from peripheral veins should be collected separately, since the variation in the amount of drug in different parts of the circulation may assist in determining how much of the poison was taken, and at what length of time before death.

If the blood is not to be taken at once to the laboratory, it should be kept in a refrigerator at about 4°C if possible, and a small amount of sodium fluoride added to prevent enzymatic decomposition of alcohol.

As regards the amount of the sample, the more that can be obtained the better, but even very small samples may be valuable, since modern methods for the analysis of alcohol, CO, etc., and for blood grouping require only very small amounts.

CHAPTER 15
Wounds

Laws of Wounding

Offences Against Person Act 1861

The offences named range from assault, even if only by a threatening gesture, and battery, when a blow is struck, to causing actual bodily harm, or grievous bodily harm, or unlawful wounding, and to manslaughter or murder when the victim dies as a result of the injury. Thus a doctor may find himself required to examine a living person with an injury, or the body of a person who has died from wounds.

The difference between murder and manslaughter is one of intent. Wounding a person with intent to kill or cause grievous bodily harm so that he dies, constitutes murder. Wounding a person so as to cause his death without such intent, e.g. during a brawl or chastisement, would constitute manslaughter.

Homicide Act 1957

This divided the crime of murder into two categories, capital murder, for which the punishment was death, and non-capital murder, punishable by imprisonment.

Capital murder comprised murder during course of theft, by shooting, and of police or prison officers while resisting arrest.

At the present, of course, the death penalty is in abeyance, and it is unlikely that it will be restored.

Suicide Act 1961

By this Act a person who commits or attempts to commit

suicide is no longer guilty of any crime. On the other hand a person who assists another to commit suicide, such as the surviving partner of a suicide pact, is guilty of manslaughter.

External injuries

Bruises

These are the result of blows with blunt objects rupturing small blood vessels, with bleeding into the adjacent tissues. The bleeding may continue for some time after the blow has been struck, and it is likely to be greater in amount in children, old people, women and anyone suffering from deficiency diseases or haematological disorders. Therefore the size of the bruise is unreliable as an indication of the amount of force causing it. Moreover, although the striking object will have had a shape, this will not be reproduced by the bruise because the continued bleeding will blur the outlines unless death occurs almost immediately after the blow, before the blood has spread far into the surrounding tissue.

As a bruise gets older it changes colour, due to alteration of the haemoglobin in the extravasated blood, passing from brown, through green to yellow. Thus fresh bruises can be distinguished from bruises a week or more old, but when examining any particular bruise it is impossible to give the precise age. Bruises are common injuries and are frequently found after fights, falls and road accidents, but they are especially significant when found on the neck, suggesting throttling (see p. 142) and on the thighs of a woman, suggeting rape (see p. 89). They can occur as post-mortem injuries, produced by forcible blows in areas of hypostasis, e.g. the back of the scalp if the body is dropped on the ground, or on trolleys or p.m. tables.

Abrasions (grazes)

These are produced by a rough surface striking the body tangentially and removing part of the outer layer of the skin.

These injuries do not blur with the passage of time unless by healing and therefore are likely to retain a clear imprint of the surface of the object which caused them, if this has a recognisable pattern. Thus they may be of great value to the pathologist when they are found on a dead body. The tread of vehicle tyres, the patterns of belts and ropes and finger-nails on the neck, and of clothing on the body may all be faithfully reproduced. A more irregular surface, such as the road, cannot leave a clear pattern but may indicate its nature by fragments of grit, etc., embedded in the raw surface of the abrasion. The direction taken by the object across the skin surface is indicated by partially detached layers of skin at the margin of the wound where the object left the skin, and by deeper linear scratches across the wound surface (figure 7).

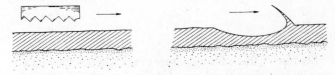

FIG. 7

After death abrasions dry and their surface is liable to become dark brown and leathery, exaggerating their apparent severity, and misleading the unwary.

Lacerations (*split wounds*)

These are produced when a blunt object strikes the skin with sufficient force to stretch and tear it. Such wounds are commonly seen in severe crushing injuries such as occur in road accidents, and may then occur anywhere on the body. When produced by falls or blows with a weapon they are usually found in situations where the skin is easily split over bone lying close beneath it, as in the scalp or eyebrows. The object causing a lacerated wound crushes and stretches a broad area of skin which then splits in its centre. Therefore the tissues at the margins of the split are grazed and bruised, and the edges of the wound are irregular, with strands of tougher tissue such as nerves or blood vessels stretching across the depths of the wound from one margin to the other (figure 8). When the bone is very close beneath the surface, as in the scalp, the margins of the wound may appear superficially to be clean cut, suggesting an incised wound, and close inspection will be necessary to determine its true nature.

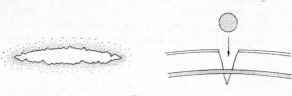

FIG. 8

Because of the splitting nature of the wounds they do not usually reproduce the shape of the striking object. However, fragments from its surface, such as coal dust, may be found buried in the wound.

These injuries cause true breaches of the skin, and are thus associated with bleeding, but this is less than might be expected from the size of the wound, since blood vessels are bruised and torn, and thus retract, and the blood clots readily.

Incised wounds (cuts)

These are cut or slashed wounds caused by sharp-edged agents, such as knives or razors. Since the agent is drawn across the body surface the wound is long, but shallow in relation to its length and is deeper at the end where the cut starts. The sharp-edged nature of the agent means that skin adjacent to the wound margin is not damaged, i.e. bruised

or abraded, and the wound edges are clean cut (figure 9).
The severed blood vessels bleed profusely.

The nature of the agent cannot be deduced from the
wound, apart from the fact that it has a sharp cutting edge.
Such wounds may be found on the neck, head and wrists in
homicidal or suicidal attempts.

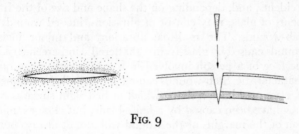

FIG. 9

Stab-wounds

These are penetrating injuries, whose depth within the body
is much greater than the size of the wounds on the body
surface. They can, of course, be produced by any long thin
object which can be thrust into the body, but almost always
are caused by knives. Therefore they have the same characteristics of clean-cut undamaged edges as incised wounds,
and usually appear as small slits. They can be mistaken for
trivial injuries because their great depth is not apparent.
Moreover, they often cause little external bleeding, most of
the haemorrhage occurring within the body cavities.

Unlike incised injuries, stab-wounds may give an indication of the shape of the weapon causing them. Thus the
overall shape of the wound will generally be elliptical, but
the ends of the wound may be pointed or rounded, as the
edges of the blade are sharp or blunt. It may also be possible
to get some idea of the dimensions of the blade from the
depth of the wound and the length of the breach in the skin,
but such measurements must never be regarded as precise,
since an exact allowance cannot be made for the elastic

E

recoil of the skin and subcutaneous tissues, nor for any part of the blade which may have remained outside the body.

Glass injuries

Damage caused by glass is not uncommon, especially in road accidents, and, depending on the shape and size of the fragments of glass, may consist of abrasions, incised wounds or stab-wounds. The multiple abrasions and minor incised wounds caused by glass from a shattered windscreen striking the face of a person involved in a road accident are quite characteristic. Stab-wounds caused accidentally by fragments of glass may have a shape which at first sight suggests that they have been caused by a knife-blade, but close examination of the margins of the wound will almost always reveal tiny side cuts due to irregularities of the glass and fragments of glass may be found embedded in the depths of the wound.

The interpretation of wounds

When confronted by a dead body bearing wounds the doctor will have to try to determine two things:

1 The nature of the agent or agents causing the injuries.
2 The circumstances in which the wounds occurred, i.e. accident, suicide or homicide.

The nature of the agent

This can often be deduced from the nature of the wounds themselves, as suggested above, e.g. bruises, abrasions and lacerations are caused by blunt objects, such as the ground, fists, hammers, clubs, etc., incised and stab-wounds by thin sharp-edged agents, e.g. knives, razor blades, spikes, etc. Abrasions may bear the pattern of the striking surface, a stab-wound will reproduce to a certain extent the shape of the blade, lacerations may show the pattern of the agent and have fragments from its surface embedded in the wound margin.

The circumstances

These can often be decided, partly from the nature of the injuries, and partly from their distribution. Each individual case has to be judged on its merits, as no two cases are exactly alike, but examples of the probable findings are:

Suicidal. The injuries are usually incised or stab-wounds, rarely bruises or abrasions. There are usually numerous injuries varying in severity from minor 'tentative' wounds scarcely penetrating the skin, to large and fatal injuries. It is possible for a suicidal wound, e.g. a stab or incised wound, to be solitary, but more commonly such wounds are multiple, and grouped in particular 'target' areas of the body, such as the neck, the wrists, the front of the chest on the left side. All the injuries must be in sites accessible to self-infliction.

Homicidal. Any type of injury from a bruise to a stab-wound may be found, and often the body of the victim bears several types of injury. Usually the injuries are all alike in severity and 'tentative' wounds are absent. If a single homicidal wound is present, distinction from suicide or accident may be difficult, or impossible, unless such a wound occurs in a site which is inaccessible to self-infliction, e.g. a stab-wound in the middle of the back could hardly be self-inflicted.

Accident. The type and distribution of injuries do not follow any particular pattern. Ususally these cases are distinguished by the attendant circumstances, or the various injuries are altogether too gross to have been either self-inflicted or due to attack by another person, e.g. a crushed head in a vehicle accident.

Example of the distinction—cut throat

Suicidal. The wound is arranged symmetrically across the front of the neck, with irregular margins caused by repeated cuts in the same area and with tentative scratches on the skin of the neck above and below the main wound. Other groups of cuts, some trivial and others deep, are likely to be found on the wrists.

Homicidal Most often a single, deep cut, asymmetrically situated at the side of the neck. There are no tentative scratches, but deep cuts are present on the face, and also on the forearms and fingers (the latter being defence injuries caused by grasping or warding off the knife).

Accident. A single deep irregular wound with gross damage to the neck structures, fracture of the cervical spine, and with multiple fractures, lacerations and abrasions elsewhere on the body.

Internal injuries

The wounds on the surface of the body are important as indicating where and how the blows fell, and why they were sustained. But, of course, they are not usually the cause of the death, which is due to internal injuries. The following are notes on some of the commoner injuries encountered in medico-legal work.

Head injuries

The head is particularly the site for impacts with hard surfaces as in falls or vehicle accidents or blows with blunt objects, e.g. fists, clubs. The commonest surface injury is likely to be a laceration of the scalp.

Skull fractures

Fractures are common after such injuries, though severe and fatal intra-cranial injury may occur without the skull having been broken. The fractures are usually fissured, either single or in a cobweb pattern, depending on the amount of force. Depressed fractures may occur if an impact with a small area, e.g. hammer-head, occurs, and these may indicate the nature of the weapon from their shape. Fractures of the base of the skull are common, especially from the severe forces encountered in vehicle accidents, and may be caused by force transmitted along the spine in falls on the feet or buttocks.

Intra-cranial haemorrhage

Extra-dural. Such a haemorrhage is liable to occur after a violent impact on the head, producing a fracture of the temporal region of the skull, with laceration of the middle meningeal artery as it lies in a groove in the bone. Rarely such haemorrhage may occur after a blow without a fracture of the skull, and it may be bilateral.

The particular medico-legal importance of this type of haemorrhage lies in the fact that, although treatable, there is considerable danger of its being overlooked. The impact which initiates the bleeding will usually cause temporary unconsciousness, but this is characteristically followed by a period of normal consciousness, the 'lucid interval', of one or more hours' duration, followed in turn by a recurrence of unconsciousness, due to rising intra-cranial pressure, and leading to death. If the patient is seen during the 'lucid interval', the doctor may not appreciate the gravity of the situation. A smell of alcohol in the patient's breath may suggest that his condition is entirely due to intoxication, with the result that he is detained in a police cell, deepening unconsciousness is mistaken for a drunken sleep, and within a few hours the patient dies.

For the safety, both of the patient and the doctor, any person who has suffered a head injury should have an X-ray examination of the skull, especially if there was a period of unconsciousness immediately after the injury, and if there is the slightest doubt about the patient's condition, even if the skull is not fractured, he should be kept under observation, and not allowed to be detained in a cell or to go home.

Sub-dural. These may occur from relatively slight impacts, often insufficient to cause unconsciousness and usually not producing fractures of the skull. They are particularly liable to have a slow course, first producing symptoms weeks or months after the original injury. They may occur after fights or falls, and are especially likely to be found in alcoholics and in children.

Sub-arachnoid. These occur most commonly from the spontaneous rupture of an aneurysm of one of the basal cerebral arteries, but occasionally trauma to the head may be responsible for the rupture. It is frequently impossible to demonstrate the actual source of bleeding at autopsy. A blow on the side of the neck can rupture the vertebral artery at the base of the skull and cause a fatal sub-arachnoid haemorrhage from blood tracking upwards from the site of the rupture. Sub-arachnoid bleeding may also occur after severe brain injury, contusion or laceration. Massive haemorrhage proves rapidly fatal.

Brain Damage

Blows to the head may cause bruising of the brain, both beneath the point of impact, and also at the opposite side of the head (contre-coup injury). The latter may be found at the front and sides of the head but not at the back. The actual mechanism is uncertain; there are several theories.

Greater force may cause actual laceration of the brain tissue. Haemorrhages within the brain may occur along the line of force, and may subsequently rupture on to the brain surface or into the ventricles. Such internal haemorrhages are especially dangerous when they occur in the brain stem, where they may cause rapid death from pressure on the vital centres.

Oedema of the brain may develop after head injury and may occur either localised to injured areas, or generally throughout the brain, causing prolonged unconsciousness or death.

The cause of concussion is unknown, but prolonged periods of unconsciousness after head injury, e.g. several weeks, have been found to be associated with partial demyelination.

Facial injuries

The fragile facial bones are particularly liable to damage from blows, either in vehicle accidents, or in fights, from blows with fists, or kicks. Characteristically fractures extend horizontally across the face through the orbits or across the upper jaw, and vertically downwards, from the orbits, often separating the middle third of the face from the outer two-thirds. The lower jaw may be broken in the centre, or near either angle. These injuries may prove rapidly fatal due to obstruction of the air passages by blood.

Neck

Damage of the neck structures is usually found in cases of strangulation (see p. 141). Severe injuries may occur in incised wounds, suicidal cut-throat, where all the tissues may be divided down to the spine. Blows on the neck may cause rupture of the trachea with rapid onset of subcutaneous emphysema. The cervical spine may be fractured —in road accidents, due to sudden jerks of the head, at the atlanto-axial joint, or in the region of the sixth cervical vertebra.

Chest

This is pre-eminently a site for stab-wounds, which usually cause death by massive intra-thoracic haemorrhage, the weapon having pierced the heart, the aorta, the pulmonary artery, or the venae-cavae. Stab-wounds of the lungs are not usually fatal, although pneumothorax occurs, unless a major pulmonary blood vessel has been severed, with consequent haemorrhage. Stab-wounds of the heart are dangerous, but if the left ventricle is pierced, the thickness of the muscle wall may restrict the bleeding, allowing sufficient time for surgical treatment. A stab of the right ventricle is more rapidly fatal, blood escaping through the wound to cause haemopericardium and cardiac tamponade.

Severe impacts on the chest, as in road accidents, may fracture ribs or cause crushing injury of the lungs, with multiple small sub-pleural emphysematous blebs, or laceration of the tissue, either of the pleural surface, or confined to the interior of the lung.

In gross crushing injuries the heart may be lacerated. Uncommonly it may be bruised, but if such bruising affects a coronary artery, it may cause a traumatic coronary thrombosis within a few hours. Traumatic rupture of the aorta commonly occurs at the junction of the arch and descending parts, just beyond the origin of the left subclavian artery, and is due to violent compression of the chest. It is common in road accidents.

Fractures of the spine may be due to flexion or extension, and are usually associated with extensive injuries elsewhere.

Abdomen

This also is a frequent site for stab-wounds, with massive haemorrhage often resulting from perforation of the aorta or other large vessels. Alternatively transfixion of the stomach or loops of bowel may cause peritonitis.

Blows may rupture the spleen, liver or kidneys, with

severe haemorrhage. More severe crushing injuries may produce gross disintegration of these organs, and rupture of hollow viscera, such as the stomach, bladder or bowel. A particular danger of such abdominal injuries is that there frequently are no signs of damage to the abdominal wall, e.g. bruising, to suggest the gravity of the condition.

Limbs

Lower limb injuries are frequent in accidents, notably of the upper leg in occupants of vehicles, and the lower leg in pedestrians (bumper-bar fracture).

Cuts, bruises or stabs may be found on the hands or arms of victims of homicidal attacks as defence injuries from attempting to ward off blows. Their severity and irregular distribution will distinguish them from suicidal injuries, with planned sites and variation in severity.

Fractures of the neck of the femur are a common result of falls by elderly people, either due to impact with the ground, or to muscle violence when falling. These cause immobility and so predispose to death from pneumonia or venous thrombosis with pulmonary embolism.

Fractures are also associated with the hazard of fat or bone marrow embolism.

CHAPTER 16
Firearms

Elementary ballistics

Firearms may be considered, in the simplest form, to be of two main types, i.e.:

1 Guns firing single missiles—rifles and pistols.
2 Guns firing a mass of small missiles, or shot—shot-guns.

Rifles and pistols

These are also known as rifled weapons, after the rifling or spiral grooving of the inside of the barrel, designed to impart a spin to the missile or bullet, and so to ensure a steady flight by the gyroscopic effect produced.

Weapons with a long barrel, 2–3 ft long, are known as rifles. These are designed to fire the missile at a very high speed, or muzzle velocity, about 1,000–4,000 ft/sec, and are accurate at a considerable range.

Short-barrelled weapons, 1–12 in long, are known as pistols, have a low muzzle velocity, 600–1,000 ft/sec, and are only accurate at relatively short range. Pistols are of two types, revolvers and automatics.

Revolvers (figure 10, left) are so called because the ammunition is put in chambers in a metal cylinder which revolves before each shot to bring the next live round opposite the barrel, ready to be fired. After the bullet has been discharged the cartridge case, the brass case which contained the explosive, remains in the cylinder, and must be removed by hand.

An automatic (or self-loading pistol) (figure 10, right) has the ammunition stored in a magazine, usually in the butt or handle of the gun, from where each round is fed into the barrel by a spring when the previous round has been fired. The empty cartridge case from the round that has been fired is *automatically* ejected from the pistol, landing on the ground several feet away.

The size or calibre of all these weapons is expressed as the internal diameter of the barrel, e.g. ·303 inches for a rifle and ·45 inches for a large pistol.

The missiles for these weapons consist of a solid metal bullet, often with a lead centre which may have a harder metal jacket. The bullet is fitted into the neck of a metal (often brass) container, the cartridge case, which contains the explosive to fire the bullet from the gun, and also a detonator, in a small copper or brass disc in the base of the cartridge case, which on being struck by the hammer released by the trigger of the gun, detonates the main part of the explosive.

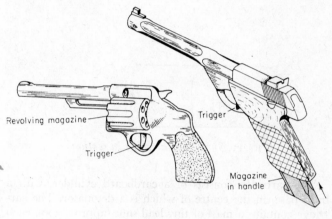

Revolving magazine

Trigger

Trigger

Magazine in handle

FIG. 10

Most of these guns have a safety catch, a device which can lock the firing mechanism and prevent the gun being discharged accidentally.

Shot-guns

These are made for shooting game; the inside of the barrel is smooth, and the gun is designed to fire a composite missile consisting of a mass of tiny lead pellets or 'shot'.

The cartridges are loaded into the weapon by hand, and the empty cases are retained in the gun after they have been fired. The guns may have one or two barrels, side by side, or over and under, and one or two triggers, one for each barrel. There are rarely any safety-catches on hammered guns, but often on hammerless weapons.

The size or calibre may either be expressed as the inside diameter of the barrel, e.g. ·410 shot-gun, or by an archaic measurement, the bore, e.g. 12-bore shot-gun. This refers to the number of balls of lead, exactly fitting the barrel, which could be made from a pound of lead.

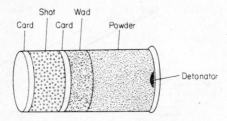

FIG. 11. *Shot-gun cartridge in section.*

The cartridge consists of a cardboard cylinder, with a brass base, in the centre of which is a detonator. The cartridge contains a mass of tiny lead shot (approx. 300), each about $\frac{1}{8}$ inch diameter, held in place by cardboard discs. At the bottom of the cylinder is the explosive powder, and between it and the shot is a thick cardboard disc, or wad, which functions as a piston, driving the shot before it down the gun barrel.

The shot leave the gun barrel as a solid mass, but gradually fan out during their passage through the air, so that the effect of the shot at close range is of one solid missile, at a few yards it is of a solid missile surrounded by several separate shot, and at greater distances, it is of many separate individual shot. The cardboard discs and the wad leave the gun with the shot, and travel for several feet before falling to the ground. Therefore in injuries caused at close range they may be found in the wound with the mass of shot.

Air-guns

These are common as adolescents' weapons, and may be of rifle or pistol type. The propellant is compressed air and the missile is a metal pellet or dart. Such weapons can be dangerous or even lethal at short ranges. Some weapons use cartridges of liquid CO_2 as the propellant, and in external appearance resemble very closely the normal revolver or automatic pistol.

Humane killers

These are specially designed for veterinary purposes for killing cattle. They may use ammunition just like normal pistols, or may be of the captive bolt type in which a metal spike is shot out of the muzzle by a blank cartridge for a few inches before being arrested.

Statutory Regulations

Firearms Act 1968

Before buying a rifled weapon, i.e. a rifle or pistol, or ammunition for such a weapon, the purchaser must have a firearms certificate, obtainable from the local chief constable. The certificate relates to a particular weapon, and a variation of the certificate must be obtained for each firearm purchased.

The authority for possession of shot-guns is a shot-gun certificate, obtained in the same way as a firearm certificate, but not relating to a particular weapon.

Air Guns do not require certificates, but it is an offence to give an air-gun to a person under the age of 14, and it is illegal for a person under 17 years to have an air-gun in a public place, unless it is protected by a gun cover.

It is an offence to shorten the barrel of a shot-gun.

Firearm wounds

Bullet wounds

These are produced by a single missile travelling at high velocity. As the bullet enters the body it generally produces a round hole with clean-cut skin edges, slightly smaller than the bullet. While the missile is travelling through the body shock waves are caused, which spread laterally into the tissues, producing a large cavity in the track of the missile several times larger than the diameter of the bullet. This cavity only persists for a fraction of a second and the track of the missile within the body will be represented by a broad band of damaged tissue. The bullet will be slowed by its passage through the tissues so that if it leaves the body its exit wound will usually be an irregular split in the skin with everted edges, rather than a clean-cut hole.

The entrance wound may have special features, dependent on the distance between the muzzle and the body when the gun is fired, e.g.:

1 Muzzle pressed against skin (contact injury). The gases produced by the explosion of the cartridge will enter through the skin with the missile and if they meet underlying bone, e.g. the skull, may be reflected, everting and splitting the skin at the margins of the entrance wound to produce a cruciform-shaped tear. The tissue at the margin of the wound may contain soot and powder, and carbon monoxide derived from the gases. The recoil of the gun barrel may produce a circular bruise on the skin beside the entrance wound.

2 Close range, i.e. 1 in–2 ft. The products of explosion, i.e. the flame, soot and particles of unburnt powder, escaping from the muzzle with the missile will mark the skin around the entrance wound with a ring of blackening by soot and tattooing by fragments of unburnt powder driven into the skin. Hair may be singed.

3 Longer range, i.e. more than 2 ft. The gun is now too

far from the skin for the products of explosion to produce any marks. Therefore, the characteristics of the entrance wound are entirely due to the bullet. As the latter penetrates the skin it inverts and abrades the margins. Therefore subsequently the wound will appear as a round hole with a band of abrasion around the margin of the hole, about $\frac{1}{16}$ in broad, and outside the abrasion a rim of soiling of the skin by grease, derived from the surface of the bullet, since bullets are packed in grease as a preservative.

Thus the range of discharge of a rifled weapon can usually be determined when it is fired close to the body, but not at any range beyond about 2 ft.

The characteristic features of the entrance wound will usually enable it to be distinguished from the exit wound, which presents as an irregular split of the skin, with everted margins, and with no soiling of the adjacent tissues by the products of explosion. Such a distinction may be important in indicating the circumstances of the shooting; thus a contact entrance wound at the front of the head, with an exit wound at the back is consistent with suicide. A close-range entrance wound at the back of the head, with an exit wound in the forehead, on the other hand, suggests the possibility of homicide.

Shot-gun wounds

Unlike bullet wounds, it is rare for there to be an exit wound, as the shot tend to scatter within the body. The track of the missile or mass of shot within the body is broader and more ragged than is the case with a bullet.

The nature of the entrance wound varies with the range:

1   *Contact injury.* If the muzzle is applied to the forehead, or the roof of the mouth, the greater part of the head, including the actual entrance wound, may be destroyed.

On the trunk the wound will present as a rounded hole, with a very narrow rim of blackening by soot at the skin edges. Soot, powder and carbon monoxide will contaminate the tissues at the margins of the wound, beneath the skin.

Recoil of the gun barrel may graze or bruise the skin beside the entrance wound.

2   *At close range,* up to 1 yard, there may still be gross destruction of the head.

Elsewhere, the shot will enter the body as a solid mass, producing a round or oval hole about 1 in diameter, with slightly ragged margins and with considerable blacking of the surrounding skin by soot and singeing of hair by flame unless the wound is produced through clothing. At this range the cards and wad from the cartridge will be blown into the wound along with the shot.

3   *At intermediate ranges*—about 1–4 yards—the bulk of the shot will still be travelling as a composite mass, but some individual shot pellets around the periphery will have begun to diverge. Thus the wound will appear as a central hole, with several tiny separate holes each up to $\frac{1}{8}$ in diameter, in the skin around the margin. There will be no naked eye evidence of soiling by soot or powder at this range, although traces may be found on swabs taken from the area of the wound. Cards and wad may be found in the wound.

4   *At long range*—over 4 yards. As the range increases the shot will become increasingly separated and the wound at more than 10 yards range approximately, will consist of a mass of separate tiny holes due to individual shot. Such a wound is, of course, only fatal when a shot has, for instance, punctured a main blood vessel, e.g. in the neck.

A rough indication of the range of discharge can be obtained by measuring the diameter of the wound, from the outermost of the individual pellet wounds, in inches, and subtracting one, when the result will indicate the range in yards, e.g. wound 6 in diameter, range 5 yards. This should only be used for a very rough estimate, since individual weapons vary considerably, and for greater accuracy test firings with the weapon must be made (see below).

Human killer wounds

These may look very similar to pistol wounds, but will have a distinct circular pattern on the skin around the periphery of the hole in the entrance wound, due to the way in which the muzzle of the gun is shaped to prevent it slipping on an animal's head.

Air-gun wounds

The pellet produces a tiny hole like the individual shot from a shot-gun. However close the range, there will be of course no soiling by soot or powder. The wounds are usually not fatal, but may be so in a child, or if the pellet injures a large blood vessel. Although rarely fatal they are liable to produce severe injuries, e.g. the loss of an eye.

The interpretation of firearm injury

From external examination

Th object, of course, primarily, is to distinguish between homicide, suicide and accident. For this, note must be taken of:

1 The probable type of weapon which caused the injury.
2 The site of the wound.
3 The range of discharge.

Thus, in the case of suicide, the wound must be capable of self-infliction, from its site (classically in the temple, forehead or mouth or over the heart) and the range of discharge (which must be at a range at which the deceased could reach the trigger unless some gadget has been devised to fire the gun from a distance).

In the case of homicide, the wounds may also be in such situations, but often they are in odd sites such as the neck or the back of the body, and at longer range. They may be multiple.

An accidental shooting may of course be by the deceased or by another, and has no features distinctive of accident. Such a case must be determined by exclusion of homicide and suicide, and by the attendant circumstances.

From autopsy

The object of the examination in addition to inspection of the surface wounds is to ascertain the direction of the missile track within the body, and the precise cause of death, and to recover the missile if this is in the body. The latter must be recovered undamaged.

A bullet may have scratches on its surface which have been produced by the barrel of the gun, and which are characteristic of that gun, so that comparison of the bullet recovered from the body with bullets fired from various weapons will enable the forensic scientist to identify the gun which was used. Similarly a cartridge case bears marks produced by the firing mechanism from which it is possible to identify the gun from which it was fired.

Therefore it is very important that all such objects, especially the missile during its removal from the body, should be treated very carefully, to avoid altering or erasing the surface markings, e.g. the ends of forceps should be wrapped in gauze before the missile is gripped.

In the case of shot-gun wounds, the cards or wads, and as much shot as possible must be collected, to determine the type of cartridge used.

If the missile cannot be easily found, then much time is saved by having the body X-rayed, since a bullet can change direction on hitting bone and end up in some very remote part of the body.

By ancillary investigations

These do not come within the province of the average doctor, but it is as well that he should know of their existence, lest he destroy the evidence vital to someone else.

Clothing. This may obviously modify the appearance of an entrance wound by trapping the soot and other products of explosion from a close-range discharge before they can reach the skin. Forensic science examination will detect them.

Discharge traces on skin. When a gun is fired some chemical traces from the discharge may be blown onto the hand holding it, and lead and nitrates may be detected by tests on swabs taken from the skin of the hand. This obviously may be useful in confirming a probable case of suicide. Therefore, the deceased's body must not be washed before these tests have been made.

Suspected weapon. Any gun found at the scene of death which could have produced the injuries will have to be examined for finger-prints and evidence of recent discharge. Furthermore the condition of the gun, e.g. well or badly maintained, and whether it is liable to accidental discharge from faulty mechanism, may be of value in determining the circumstances of the death.

Range of discharge. In cases of shot-gun injuries particularly, the range of discharge can be determined fairly accurately if the weapon is available, by firing at cardboard targets at different distances and comparing the shot patterns with the wound on the body. This allows for individual variation of weapon and ammunition, which is not possible from examination of the wound alone.

CHAPTER 17
Asphyxia

Definitions

Many students tend to use the words asphyxia and anoxia without being clear as to their meaning.

Anoxia means a lack of oxygen. Four different causes for this deficiency have been described (Camps and Purchase), i.e. Anoxic anoxia—oxygen cannot reach the blood, because there is a lack of oxygen in the lungs. Anaemic anoxia—blood cannot absorb oxygen, e.g. carbon monoxide poisoning. Stagnant anoxia—blood cannot carry oxygen to tissues, e.g. heart failure or embolism. Histotoxic anoxia— the tissues cannot take up oxygen, e.g. cyanide poisoning.

The last three conditions are likely to be due to natural disease or to various poisons. The first, anoxic anoxia, due to lack of oxygen in the inspired air, or mechanical obstruction to respiration, is usually known as asphyxia, or mechanical asphyxia. This is the subject of this chapter and is dealt with under various headings:

Suffocation
Choking
Crush asphyxia
Hanging
Strangulation

It must be remembered that in these various forms of mechanical asphyxia simple lack of oxygen is not the only, nor necessarily the most important factor. CO_2 accumulation may be equally disastrous, as may various cardio-vascular disturbances. Together these produce the characteristic signs of asphyxia, i.e. congestion and engorgement, both externally and internally, especially of the face, with cyanosis and multiple petechial haemorrhages, most noticeable on the eyelids and skin of the face, due to rupture of capillaries from oxygen lack and raised blood pressure. The time taken for these various signs to occur depends on the circumstances, from a few seconds to several minutes.

These changes may sometimes be absent in circumstances otherwise suggestive of asphyxia, due to the occurrence of abrupt cardiac arrest (cardiac inhibition).

Cardiac inhibition

This may be a factor causing or contributing to death in any of the different kinds of mechanical asphyxia, but notably strangulation. A stimulus, such as compression, to any sensitive area, e.g. the larynx, a bronchus, or the vagus nerve itself in the neck, triggers off nerve impulses via the parasympathetic vagus nerve to the heart, which exceed the normal function of slowing the heart rate, and cause abrupt cardiac arrest. When the stimulus is associated with obstruction of the air passages, death occurs suddenly before there has been time for the normal processes of asphyxia, and their diagnostic signs, to develop.

Cardiac inhibition may occur in conditions other than mechanical asphyxia, e.g. in abortion, from blows to the abdomen, drowning, etc., in fact in any circumstances where violent stimulation of the parasympathetic nervous system can be caused.

Autopsy may reveal signs of the initiating cause, e.g. strangulation, but obviously cannot demonstrate the actual mechanism, which is a physiological process, by anatomical means. Diagnosis will depend on exclusion of other causes of death, and a consideration of the circumstances.

Suffocation

Death will occur if there is insufficient oxygen in the local atmosphere. Such circumstances are usually the imprisonment of the victim in a small unventilated space, e.g. in a coal mine after a roof fall, in a large safe or refrigerator, etc.

In the course of time oxygen is used up, and replaced by CO_2, and death probably occurs from the combined effects of anoxia and CO_2 narcosis and possibly heat and injuries. Under these circumstances death usually occurs only after several hours and the signs of asphyxia, i.e. cyanosis, petechial haemorrhages, etc., are especially well developed. The time actually taken to die will depend, of course, on the size of the space and the amount of available oxygen, and the needs of the victim, i.e. if he is working or is at rest.

Smothering

In this form of asphyxia the mouth and nose are obstructed. Thus a person may become smothered by heavy bedclothes, and infants may be smothered by a hand applied to the nose and mouth, by turning face down into a soft pillow, or by being overlayed by an adult's body. Putting a plastic bag over the head may cause smothering, either accidentally, in children, or deliberately as a means of suicide, in adults. Murder may be accomplished by smothering, as by covering the face with a soft pillow, as in the story of the Princes in the Tower. It is a criminal offence for an adult, over 16, to have a child under 3 in bed with him, while he is under the influence of alcohol, because of the danger of smothering, notably overlaying.

The signs of asphyxia are usually fully developed, though death is likely to be more rapid than in suffocation; choking (see below) due to inhalation of vomit caused by anoxia may accelerate the death. On occasions when the air passages are suddenly and completely obstructed as in smothering by a plastic bag, death may in fact be due to cardiac inhibition, with no signs of asphyxia.

Homicidal smothering is always difficult to diagnose, since there will probably be no signs other than those of asphyxia. The use of an object such as a soft pillow will leave no marks or injuries to indicate the method.

Choking

Choking is caused by blockage of the air passages by foreign material. This may come from inside or outside the body.

Thus, the air passages may be blocked by inhaled vomit, by disease such as carcinoma, from falling back of the tongue during unconsciousness, or by blood or broken dentures, following facial injuries. The material may be partially masticated food, as in children or mentally defective persons, sand, flour, etc., in industrial accidents, or cotton wool, cloth, etc., in intentional choking as a means of suicide, infanticide or homicide, or as part of a gag.

Again, signs of asphyxia are likely to be well developed unless cardiac inhibition supervenes. The diagnosis is likely to be apparent from the history, i.e. a sudden attack of coughing and gasping with cyanosis ,followed by death, and confirmed by the demonstration, at autopsy, of foreign material in the air passages. Occasionally, however, death may supervene rapidly with no signs of choking, especially when death is due to cardiac inhibition from inhaling food and such cases may be suggestive of a heart attack. They have been called 'Café Coronaries'.

Crush asphyxia

Crush asphyxia is due to compression of the body or chest by some heavy weight, such as a vehicle, or soil from the sides of a trench which has collapsed. The chest is compressed and the diaphragm fixed, by compression of the abdominal wall, so that respiratory movement is impossible, and compression of the legs and abdomen forces blood into the head.

These factors produce a characteristic appearance of the

victim, comprising deep engorgement and cyanosis with many large haemorrhages in the skin of the upper part of the body from the mid-chest including the shoulders and the head, and with swelling and oedema of the eyeballs, and haemorrhages into the conjunctivae.

Hanging

Hanging is due to compression of the neck, usually by a ligature, in such a manner that the tension is determined by the weight of the whole, or part, of the victim's body.

Hanging from a high point of suspension

In this case the victim is either fully suspended, with the feet clear of the ground, or is suspended in the standing posture, the knees slightly flexed.

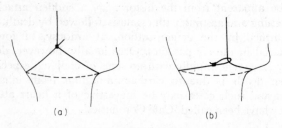

Fig. 12. *Suspension.* (a) *Fixed noose,* (b) *running noose.*

Suspension is by a ligature, usually a rope, with a noose which encircles the neck. The noose may either be fixed, when the rope is knotted, or a running noose, as when the end of the rope is passed through a loop.

The pressure of the ligature will produce a groove or complete closure of the blood vessels, notably the carotid arteries, and also the air passages, with resultant cerebral anoxia, unconsciousness occurring within seconds and death within a few minutes. Signs of asphyxia are usually absent, and the face is pale and placid.

The pressure of the ligature will produce a groove or furrow in the skin of the upper part of the neck. If the ligature has a rough surface the floor of the groove will be abraded. An imprint of the surface of the ligature may be seen.

The course of the groove will depend on whether a fixed or running noose has been used. In the case of a fixed noose the side of the noose nearest to the suspending rope will be pulled upwards, assuming the shape of an inverted V. The groove in the skin will therefore have a corresponding course often with a zone of unmarked skin at the apex of the V, caused by the head falling away from the rope.

When a running noose has been used, the weight of the body will cause the noose to tighten in a mainly horizontal position. The groove will therefore also be mainly horizontal, but there may be an additional vertical mark caused by the suspending ligature.

The internal damage to neck structures is often slight compared to the depth of the skin groove. Muscles, e.g. the sternomastoids, may be ruptured, and the hyoid bone and thyroid cartilage may be broken, but bleeding at the site of these injuries is slight or absent. If the body dropped several feet before the rope tightened the cervical spine may be dislocated at the atlanto-axial joints.

The circumstances of such suspension are usually those of suicide, and this may be confirmed by the presence of suicide notes, and of a platform, such as a chair, table, etc., used to effect the suspension. The absence of such a platform and the presence of any injuries on the body apart from the mark of the ligature should be regarded with suspicion. They may indicate that the person was killed by some other means, and the body then suspended to conceal the crime.

Hanging from a low point of suspension

A comparatively slight force, about 10 lb, is sufficient to occlude the blood vessels of the neck. Therefore a person can die from hanging even though the greater part of the body weight is supported by the ground, e.g. by suspension of the body in a crouching position from a door handle or bed-head.

The appearance of the body usually differs from that seen in hanging from a high point of suspension. The groove produced by the ligature is less well-marked, and may be lower on the neck and more nearly horizontal. The initial effect of the ligature is to occlude the veins, so that the face is swollen, purple in colour, with many petechial haemorrhages, i.e. the appearances are those of slow asphyxia.

Such a method may be used when full suspension is impracticable, e.g. in prison. However, it may also be used by persons curious to experience some of the effects of hanging, or may be a feature of sexual perversion, the victim being unaware that even partial occlusion of the blood vessels may cause rapid loss of consciousness. In the case of sexual perversion the deceased, always a male, may be naked or wearing female clothing and pornographic literature may be found at the scene. There may also be some soft padding, such as a handkerchief, between the ligature and the neck.

Hanging with incomplete encirclement of the neck

Hanging may occur when pressure is only applied to the front of the neck, e.g. by the arm of a chair, edge of a settee, rung of a ladder, etc. The circumstances of such hanging are almost always accidental. Marks on the neck may be indistinct or absent.

Strangulation

This is due to constriction of the neck by a force applied other than by the weight of the body, usually by a ligature tightened by the hands, or by the hands themselves.

Strangulation by a ligature

The ligature. This may be any strip of pliable material, but since it will need to be something which is readily to hand, is usually either a tie or a stocking. The ligature may be put round the neck and the ends crossed and pulled tight, or it may be applied and knotted. The knot is usually at the front or side and may be of any kind, but the ligature should be photographed *in situ*, and then removed by cutting, without untying the knot since if it is an unusual type it may provide the police with valuable evidence. The ligature may be removed by the assailant, and strangulation must then be deduced from the marks on the neck, and distinguished from hanging.

The ligature mark. This consists of a horizontal groove around the neck, at about the level of the thyroid cartilage. It is usually much less well-marked than a hanging mark, and if a soft ligature has been used it may be almost invisible. If the ligature has been crossed and pulled tight the mark is likely to be more prominent at the site of cross-over, where the two ends of the mark may be at different levels. If knotted, the ligature mark will be continuous, but broader at the site of the knot. The groove may bear the imprint of the surface of the ligature, and also on the neck there may be scratches or bruises caused by the hands of the assailant, or the hands of the victim when endeavouring to relieve the pressure.

It is necessary to avoid mistaking marks caused by tight clothing for ligature marks, and also the pallid marks found in skin folds in the fat necks of babies.

Signs of asphyxia, congestion and petechial haemorrhages are usually prominent in the head above the level of the ligature mark, but such signs may be absent where death is rapid, as by cardiac inhibition. Other injuries, such as lacerations of the scalp, stab-wounds or evidence of rape, may be found in homicidal strangulation.

Internal Injuries. Such damage usually consists of bruising of neck muscles and also fractures, particularly of the thyroid cartilage, at the level of the ligature, unless the victim is young, and the cartilage elastic. Above this level the soft tissues, especially lymph-nodes and the root of the tongue, will be congested. Oedema of the lungs with foam in the air passages is frequently present.

Suicidal strangulation. This is uncommon as a method of suicide. A means of applying the ligature so that it remains in position after unconsciousness occurs is required. This may be achieved by using ligatures with rough or adhesive surfaces, by multiple loose turns round the neck, by a tourniquet mechanism, etc. Signs of asphyxia are well-marked, but there is little damage to neck structures, and the ligature mark is usually only a faint band of pallor.

Accidental strangulation. In adults this is only likely to occur if clothing is caught in machinery, though it might be produced by tight clothes, e.g. collar and tie, in a person who was deeply drunk.

It is liable to happen to small children, who get entangled in pram harness or other impedimenta.

Strangulation by the hands—throttling

This form of strangulation only occurs from homicidal attempts because in attempted self-throttling, unconsciousness would cause the hands to loosen their grip. The neck may be gripped by one or both hands, usually from the front. The external findings are bruises produced by the digits, at the front and sides of the neck, which are usually rounded and about ½ in in diameter, but may be very faint. If the asasilant has long nails these may cause scratches which present as tiny crescentic abrasions about ¼ in long. There are usually well-developed signs of asphyxia, and other injuries are likely to be present, e.g. bruises on the face, lacerations of the scalp, or signs of sexual interference.

The damage to the internal neck structures is likely to be more severe than in other forms of strangulation, since greater pressure can be applied in localised areas, e.g. by the thumb. Thus, extensive fractures of the hyoid bone or the thyroid and cricoid cartilages may be found, with localised, but severe bruising of the muscles.

The external appearances may be modified if clothing was interposed between the neck and the hands, so that in effect a partial ligature was used, and also in a rare form of strangulation, mugging, in which pressure on the neck is applied by the forearm, the assailant being behind his victim. This may leave few external signs of injury because of the broad area and soft surface of the arm.

Throttling may cause cardiac inhibition, probably due to the fact that the digits can exert localised but very deep pressure directly impinging on the vagus nerve. However, this result can also occur from less severe pressure, as by a light blow or slight squeezing of the neck.

CHAPTER 18
Drowning

The diagnosis of drowning is a fairly common medico-legal problem. A body may be recovered from water and the doctor asked to examine it with the object of ascertaining whether or not death was due to drowning. In such a case it is unsafe to rely on the fact that the deceased has been found submerged. Death may have been due to a heart attack, during which the victim fell into the water, or the person made have been killed, e.g. by strangulation, and the body then dumped in water. If the body is badly decomposed, such diagnosis may be very difficult. Moreover, in some cases drowning may not be suspected, as when it occurs in shallow water, as from immersion of a drunken man's face in a puddle.

The questions which the doctor may have to answer are:
1 Was death due to drowning, or to some other cause?
2 How long has the body been in the water?
3 What is the identity of the deceased? This problem often arises in connection with drowning since the body may drift a considerable distance from the original site of entering the water and be recovered in a region where the deceased is not known. (For methods of identification, see Chapter 23.)

Causes of death in submersion

Typical drowning

During the initial struggles some water enters the air passages, and more as the body sinks. Due to the respiratory movements the water mixes with mucus and surfactant from the lungs to make a froth in the air passages. Struggling is followed by a quiescent phase, then terminal convulsions and death.

When the water is inhaled into the lungs it will affect the blood. Fresh water, i.e. from canals, rivers, etc., which is hypotonic to plasma, will enter via the pulmonary capillaries and dilute the blood while sea-water, being hypertonic, will extract water from the blood in the pulmonary circulation, making it more concentrated. In fresh-water drowning, water to the extent of about 2 litres may be absorbed, though in a baby 30 or 40 ml may be sufficient to cause death.

Therefore death in drowning is partly due to anoxia by exclusion of air from the lungs, but principally due to electrolyte disturbance and/or haemolysis, from the effects of the inhaled water on the blood.

Cardiac inhibition

This is likely to occur in sudden total submersion in cold water, especially when this is totally unexpected, as when walking over a dock edge. Even when submersion is anticipated, e.g. at swimming-baths, a misjudged dive with sudden entry of water into the naso-pharynx may cause cardiac inhibition. Death will then occur rapidly and the normal processes of drowning will not take place.

Laryngeal spasm

This is an uncommon consequence of submersion, but entry of water into the larynx may cause severe laryngeal spasm with closure of the airway. In effect the victim dies of choking, with signs of asphyxia, which are rarely seen in typical drowning.

The appearance of the freshly drowned body

Externally the body may show signs of submersion, i.e.

sodden clothing, mud-stained and wrinkled skin, etc. Hypostasis is mainly in the head and neck. The only signs indicative of drowning as opposed to submersion are the presence
of fine, persistent, white foam at the nostrils and mouth,
more exuding if the chest is compressed, and the presence
of objects from the water, such as water-weeds, tightly
grasped in the hands by cadaveric spasm. Signs of asphyxia,
e.g. petechial haemorrhages, etc., are not usually seen. At
autopsy, the lungs will appear distended, with pallor of
their surfaces, rather like asthmatic lungs, but are heavy and
wet with large areas of purple mottling beneath the
pleuri, and pressure from a finger will leave an indentation
on the surface. The trachea and bronchi, and the cut
surfaces of the lungs will contain foamy water, though
occasionally all the water is absorbed, leaving the lungs dry.
Water may also be present in the oesophagus and stomach,
and this may contain algae or pond-weed indicating its
source. Haemolysis of the blood may be apparent and may
produce haemolytic staining of the wall of the aorta, not
seen in the pulmonary artery. These classical signs of
drowning will disappear in a few days, due to putrefaction.

Confirmatory evidence of drowning

The nature of the water in the lungs

It may be necessary to distinguish water inhaled in drowning from the serous fluid in pulmonary oedema. This may
be possible by microscopical examination of water in the
stomach or exuding from the lung surface for algae, etc., or
by maceration of fragments of lung tissue in distilled water.

Biochemical tests on blood

These seek to demonstrate dilution or concentration of the
blood to a different degree on each side of the heart. Thus
in fresh-water drowning the blood on the left side of the
heart, i.e. after passing through the lungs, will be diluted

compared with that in the right side of the heart. In salt-water drowning the reverse will occur.

Such alterations can be shown by determining the specific gravities of sera from the two sides, or by determining any of the serum electrolytes, e.g. sodium or chloride ions.

These tests are only reliable if applied within about 24–48 hours after death, before putrefactive changes have disturbed the blood chemistry.

Diatom tests

If the water entering the blood during drowning is from such natural sources as rivers or lakes, it is likely to contain diatoms, and these will be distributed throughout the body by the circulation. Organs can then be removed at autopsy and all soft tissue digested with concentrated mineral acids, leaving only the acid-resistant silica shells of the diatoms. If the diatoms are discovered in such sites as the liver, brain or bone marrow this is strong evidence of drowning and is especially valuable where putrefaction has tendered useless all the other methods of making the diagnosis. However, some natural waters contain few diatoms and moreover, there is a seasonal variation in the numbers of these microscopic plants, few being present in winter.

Injuries present on submerged bodies

Such injuries are relatively common, being caused after death by passing boats, by fish or aquatic mammals, or by bumping against rocks. When caused within a few hours after death, such injuries may show appreciable bruising, especially those of the head, possibly due to dilution and haemolysis of the blood, or to the distribution of hypostasis. Because of this, and the fact that wounds caused before death may be altered in appearance by the haemolysing action of the water, it may be very difficult in the case of external injuries on the body to decide whether they

F

were caused before or after death. There should be no such difficulty, however, in regard to internal injuries, e.g. intracranial haemorrhage, damage to neck structures from throttling, etc.

Contributory factors in drowning

The autopsy in a case of drowning should be able to demonstrate any natural disease which may have caused or contributed to submersion, e.g. heart disease, cerebral infarction, etc.

Moreover, no investigation of a drowning is complete, unless putrefaction has occurred, without at least a determination of the presence and the amount of any alcohol in the body, and the possibility that other drugs may be present must be remembered.

Determination of the period of submersion

Body temperature

Cooling is usually at approximately twice the rate in air, i.e. at about 3–4°F per hour, and the body will usually feel cold within a short time after submersion.

Skin changes

Whitening and wrinkling of the skin (notably of the palms and soles) occurs within a few hours. More slowly, over one or two weeks, the nails and hair become loosened and shed; after about two weeks the skin of the hands and feet is loosened, and may be stripped off. (Finger-prints may be taken from the separated skin of the fingers, or from the exposed dermis.)

Putrefaction

This, like all the other changes mentioned here, depends to

a large extent on the nature and temperature of the surrounding water. Bodies in water containing hot chemical effluent from factories may show gross putrefaction in 24 hours. Otherwise the changes may be slowed down, but develop rapidly when the body is removed from the water.

Adipocere

This is likely to occur in submersion, and parts or the whole of the body may be preserved. The changes are likely to take several months to become fully developed.

CHAPTER 19
Physical Agents

Heat

General effects

'*Heat stroke*'—Heat hyperpyrexia. This occurs when there is a high air temperature. The body's heat-regulating mechanism becomes overwhelmed and breaks down, especially if the usual cooling mechanisms are interfered with. The body temperature rapidly rises to 107–110°F, the victim develops convulsions and lapses into coma and may die. In reported cases a feature at autopsy was the large number of petechial haemorrhages in the internal organs, especially the brain.

This condition may occur in otherwise healthy people suddenly exposed to very high temperature, but is also a potential hazard of any drug which modifies the action of the heat-regulating mechanism, notably atropine used in premedication, especially if the patient is then exposed to a high air temperature in the theatre. A variety of malignant hyperpyrexia has recently been recognised as occurring during anaesthesia with certain agents and due to an underlying inherited myopathy.

Heat exhaustion. This is due to prolonged exposure to hot conditions, though not as hot as those producing heat stroke. If the salt and water loss from sweating is replaced by pure water, the body becomes salt deficient, and the victim develops weakness, faintness, muscle cramps, skin rashes, etc. Replacement of the salt cures the condition, and prophylactic supplies, e.g. salt tablets, will prevent it.

Local effects—burns

The effect of local exposure of the body to heat is to produce a burn the severity of which depends on the length of exposure and the temperature of the heat source. The minimum temperature capable of producing a burn is about 44°C for an exposure of about 5 to 6 hours. 2 sec is sufficient at 65°C.

Various classifications of the severity of burns are available, the simplest being of 3 degrees:

1st degree—skin reddening and blistering
2nd degree—whole skin destruction
3rd degree—damage, charring, etc., to tissues beneath the skin.

In addition to the depth of the burn, the other factor of importance is the surface area of the body which is affected. Twenty per cent involvement, even by superficial burns, is dangerous to life.

A dead body can of course be burnt as well as a live one. Post-mortem burns can be distinguished from ante-mortem injuries by the absence of reddening of the skin at the margins, the absence of significant amounts of protein in the fluid of blisters, and the absence of microscopic evidence of inflammatory reaction.

Causes of death from burns

1 Primary (neurogenic) shock—due to pain, etc.
2 Secondary (oligaemic) shock—due to fluid loss from burned surfaces.
3 Toxaemia—absorption of various metabolites from the burnt tissue.
4 Infection, local and septicaemia.
5 Biochemical disturbances, secondary to the fluid loss, and destruction of tissue, such as hypokalaemia.
6 Acute renal failure, due to lower nephron nephrosis.
7 Gastro-intestinal disturbances— acute peptic ulcerations (Curling's ulcer), dilatation of the stomach, haemorrhage into the intestine.
8 Glottic or pulmonary oedema—due to burns of the air passages, by inhalation of flame or hot gases.

The examination of a burnt body

This usually arises when a body is found in a house or vehicle which has been the seat of a fire. The same type of considerations apply as in the case of drowning, i.e. the fact that the body is burnt and at the site of a fire is not sufficient proof that death was due to burns. The person may have died naturally, before the fire, or have been murdered, and the fire started to conceal any evidence of the crime.

The cause of death

Death in a burning building may be due to:
1 Burns.
2 Poisoning by inhaling fumes, notably carbon monoxide.
3 Injuries from falling masonry, etc.

4 Natural disease, e.g. heart failure due to coronary atheroma, precipitated by fear or exertion.

The fact that death was due to the fire may be shown by:

The burns on the surface of the body. These may show vital reaction; i.e. reddening at the burn margin, microscopical evidence of vital reaction, etc. Moreover, the distribution of the burns on the body surface may help to show the seat of the fire, and the position of the deceased when the fire started.

The air passages. If the deceased was alive during the conflagration the trachea, etc., will contain particles of soot adhering to the walls or embedded in viscid mucus.

The blood. In almost all cases when the deceased was alive during the fire, the blood will contain carbon monoxide derived from the fumes, often in considerable amount, e.g. up to 80% in children. The blood should always be examined for alcohol, and in appropriate circumstance for other drugs, since the findings, e.g. drunkenness, may help to explain how the fire started.

Special damage caused by fire

In addition to burns, damage may be produced by the action of heat on the body, living or dead, and must be distinguished from injuries caused by other means.

Pugilistic attitude. The heat causes the muscles of the limbs to stiffen and contract, so that the arms become flexed and the hands clenched, the appearance suggesting that the deceased was engaged in a fight at the moment of death.

Heat ruptures. The contraction of the skin caused by the heat may make it tear, producing large ragged wounds, resembling lacerations. When present on the scalp they can easily be mistaken for ante-mortem injuries produced by blows with a weapon. Distinction may be by their position in a burned area, and the absence of vital reaction, or bleeding.

Heat haematoma. The heat causes blood to escape from the tissues into the sub-dural space, where it resembles an ante-mortem injury. It may be distinguished by its position, corresponding to the site of maximum charring of the head, and the absence of other injuries, e.g. fractures of the skull.

Concealment of a crime by arson

Examination of the body may reveal bullet wounds, stab-wounds, ligatures round the neck, etc., and no signs that the deceased was alive during the fire. It is unlikely that such evidence of crime will be destroyed unless damage by burning is very severe.

'Spontaneous combustion'

At one time the body was thought to be relatively incombustible, due to its high water content. However, experiments have shown that human fat is quite inflammable. This accounts for the occasions when a dead body, ignited at one point by a relatively small heat source, such as a domestic hearth fire, becomes almost completely consumed within a short time, though objects in close proximity to the body, e.g. furniture in a room, are not damaged. These circumstances are known as preternatural combustion. In the old days they were ascribed by the credulous to 'spontaneous combustion', or to mystical events (see Dickens' *Bleak House*).

Scalds

The production of damage by the application of hot liquids

is usually caused by accident, as when steam-pipes burst, or a child is dropped into a hot bath, or overturns a kettle. Very rarely the damage is produced deliberately, e.g. by a jealous wife, or as a means of murdering a child.

The injuries do not penetrate deeply, but may be dangerous because of the extent of body surface affected, or when affecting the upper air passages. They can be distinguished from burns by the lack of singeing of hairs.

The scald may reproduce the course taken by the hot liquid trickling over the skin, and so indicate the position of the body at the time of injury.

Cold

General effects—hypothermia

Three groups of persons are mainly at risk in this country:
1 infants
2 elderly people
3 climbers, potholers, etc.

Infants. Cold injury may be due to inadequate clothing or heating, from poverty, or ignorance, or deliberately, and is especially liable to affect small or premature infants. For full details, textbooks of pediatrics should be consulted, but in summary the child has a good colour, and does not appear ill, but is apathetic, feels cold when touched, and possibly has patches of hardening of subcutaneous tissue.

Elderly persons. These are usually living alone, with inadequate fuel or clothing, and with associated disease, e.g. myxoedema, cerebral arteriosclerosis, etc. The principal signs are pallor, mental apathy or coma, and coldness of the body. Temperatures of 90°F or less may be recorded by special low-reading thermometers. At body temperatures below 90°F shivering ceases, the victim does not feel cold, and the body temperature commences to fall progressively as bodily functions fail. Below 75°F death is almost inevitable and the body temperature falls to the level of the surroundings.

At autopsy the principal signs in such persons are those of associated diseases and senility, but changes specifically due to the hypothermia may be multiple thromboses, cerebral infarction, gastric erosions, and acute pancreatitis.

Climbers, etc. Sooner or later any persons exposed to severe weather conditions may develop hypothermia, but this will be hastened by inadequate clothing, wet and windy conditions, lack of body fat, inexperience and the consumption of alcohol. Fatigue is rapidly followed by exhaustion, coma, convulsions and death. Post-mortem findings are usually non-specific, but a striking feature may be the extreme bright pink colour of the blood, resembling that seen in carbon monoxide poisoning.

Incapacitation by injury or drugs, especially drunkenness, may cause deaths from exposure and hypothermia, even in urban areas.

Local effects

These are described as (1) Frostbite, and (2) 'Immersion foot', but these are variations of the same condition produced by varying degrees of dry or wet cold. Slowing of the circulation is followed by damage to blood vessels, exudation and oedema, and nerve injury. Blood becomes concentrated, the circulation may cease completely and gangrene develop, especially when tissue demands for oxygen are increased by rapid reheating. In 'Immersion foot' gangrene is less likely to develop, but there may be severe residual nerve and vascular damage.

Electricity

Factors in electrocution

A.C. current is the source of most fatalities and 50 cycles the most dangerous frequency.

The voltage. Most deaths are from supplies at about 240 volts, since that is the common domestic supply; voltages below 50 very rarely cause death. High voltages are of course dangerous, but may cause the victim to be thrown clear, while lower tensions, around 240, cause muscle contraction whereby the victim holds on to the source of the current.

Amperage. This is the most important factor. Currents of 10 mA cause pain and muscle contractions, over 60 mA are dangerous, and 100 mA is fatal. Currents over 4A are less dangerous, e.g. high-amperage currents are used therapeutically in defibrillators.

Resistance. This may be provided by the skin, or by clothing, e.g. footwear. Dryness increases the resistance, and therefore reduces the danger. Blood has a low resistance and hence within the body electricity tends to be conducted along blood vessels.

Earthing. Unless the victim is connected to 'earth' the current cannot flow. Therefore insulation from earth, e.g. by rubber-soled shoes, reduces the risk.

Duration of contact. Even currents of low tension may kill if the contact is prolonged.

Site of contact. Currents passing in the body across the chest, from hand to hand, or right hand to left leg, are particularly dangerous.

Causes of death

1 Ventricular fibrillation—the most important cause.
2 Respiratory failure—notably from paralysis of the muscles of respiration.
3 Central nervous system damage—usually due to contact of the source of electricity with the head.
4 Late effects—from burns or secondary haemorrhage, due to injuries caused by the current.

Post-mortem evidence

The circumstances of the death. Persons using electricity as a means of suicide will be found with wires and apparatus in position, e.g. connecting the wrists to a wall plug-socket. Accidental electrocution will usually be indicated by the position of the victims, especially when it appears that they have been making repairs to domestic appliances such as kettles, lamps, etc., or when there has been careless use of appliances, e.g. using an electric fire in a position where it can topple into a bath.

The electric mark. This is the site at which electricity enters the body and a similar mark may be found at the point of exit. Its size and distinctiveness depend on the size of the contact, the resistance of the skin, and the size of the current flowing. It usually presents as a small area of pale, hardened skin, sometimes blistered, or depressed with a raised rim, and with reddening of the adjacent skin, in fact very like a localised deep burn. If the area of contact is very large, e.g. from bath water, it is unlikely to leave any mark.

Electric burns. These are likely with very high voltages, and produce gross destruction of tissue, even charring of bone.

Internal evidence. This is likely to be sparse, and frequently non-existent. There may be damage to the walls of blood vessels along the path of the current, or petechial haemorrhages when asphyxia has played a part in the death.

Lightning stroke

Although this also is due to the passage of electricity through the body, the appearances are different because of the very high voltage, and the blast wave produced by the discharge of electricity through the air.

Evidence at post-mortem may be:

1 Burns. These may be widespread and fan-like (called arborescent markings), due to passage of electricity over the surface of the skin, or localised to the situation of metal objects, such as wrist-watches, bracelets, buckles, etc. The metal may become magnetised.

2 Wounds. There may be gross wounds caused by the blast effect, with lacerations and fractures, suggesting an explosion.

3 Clothing. This may be torn or burnt or melted (e.g. nylon) or may be completely stripped from the body. At first sight this may suggest that the victim has been assaulted. Death is not inevitable from lightning stroke, but the victim may be concussed, or require artificial respiration. Sequelae may be paralyses, or mental changes, or deafness, due to rupture of the ear-drum.

Radiation

Ultra-violet

The effects of this are familiar as sunburn. Severe damage may occur in unexpected circumstances where health lamps, or ultra-violet sterilisation are employed. Blindness from retinal damage is a possible hazard.

X-rays

These cause cell damage, or necrosis, and damage to blood vessels. High dosage may have local or general effects. Local burns, followed by sloughing which is very reluctant to heal, may occur. Pigmentation and scarring may follow and a late result is skin cancer.

General effects include sterility, aplastic anaemia, and deformities of the foetus *in utero*. Internal organs may develop necrosis or fibrosis, especially the kidneys (radiation nephritis).

Atomic radiation

The immediate effects of atomic explosion are intense heat and blast waves, causing burns and injuries. The effects of the damage to cells of the body produced by radiation may be 'radiation sickness', with vomiting, diarrhoea and haemorrhage occurring within a few days of exposure, or the later development of leukaemia or cachexia. The offspring of affected persons may show congenital abnormalities due to damage of the foetus *in utero*, or of the parents' germinal tissue, or sterility may develop in persons exposed to radiation.

CHAPTER 20
Deprivation—Starvation and Neglect

Starvation

In this country such a cause of death in adults is rare, unlike other less developed parts of the world where famine conditions occur, if crops fail. The circumstances in which a doctor is likely to see a case are:

(a) As a consequence of disease preventing the taking of food, i.e. carcinoma of the oesophagus.

(b) In self-neglect by the aged or mentally ill, whether from lack of money or understanding of the necessity of food.

(c) As a result of accidental entombment, e.g. in a colliery accident.

(d) From neglect of children or mental defectives by their parents or guardians, whether deliberately or from ignorance.

Effects of starvation

The effects of starvation depend to a certain extent on whether water is available or not. If both water and food are unavailable, death will occur in 7–10 days. If water is available, life may continue for as long as 60 days, but once 60% of the body weight has been lost, then death is almost inevitable.

The absence of food means that the body must consume its own tissues, notably protein to supply energy, and that no vitamins are available. The victim becomes emaciated, with progressive cardiac failure and with oedema and effusions into body spaces due to reduction of the plasma proteins. Frequency of urine and ketonuria occur, and there are signs of vitamin deficiency such as beriberi, pellagra, etc. Lowered resistance leads to terminal infections, bronchopneumonia, tuberculosis, typhus, etc.

Findings at autopsy

The most striking features are emaciation of the body with almost total absence of subcutaneous or intra-abdominal fat. All the organs will be reduced in size and the walls of the intestines are very thin, while the gall-bladder is distended by bile. There may be necrosis of the liver, though probably only detectable microscopically, and signs of a terminal infection.

Neglect and cruelty

In the vast majority of cases this is a matter of neglect of children by their parents or guardians. It may take the form of:
1 Insufficient cleanliness, clothing, warmth.
2 Lack of food, or unsuitable food.
3 Mental cruelty.
4 Physical violence.

The interpretation and investigation of such a case is extremely difficult, one of the most complicated problems in forensic medicine. The doctor has a dual role, in the early recognition and treatment among his patients, and in the examination, either of a living child, alleged to be the victim of cruelty, or of a child found dead in suspicious circumstances.

He must be extremely cautious before imputing lack of clothing, malnutrition, dirtiness, to deliberate neglect on the part of the parents. Small babies in particular may be below the normal weight for their age due to feeding problems arising from ignorance on the part of the mother, or weight loss may be due to natural disease, or the wrong type of food. Children quickly soil and damage clothes and poor families may not be able to replace them fast enough. Also children bruise easily and may sustain several surface injuries in the course of a day's play, so that the appearance of a thin, dirty, bruised, ragged child may be far more suggestive of wilful neglect than is in fact the case.

The most definite suggestion of deliberate cruelty is likely to occur when the child is found to be suffering from a severe injury, and this is when the child is likely to be first seen by the doctor. The occurrence of such cases has led to the definition of the 'Battered Baby' syndrome.

Battered Baby Syndrome

This was first described in America by a radiologist, Caffey, in 1946; the number of cases appears to have increased rapidly over the last few years.

The usual situation is that a child is brought in with some condition, a useless swollen arm, for instance. An X-ray demonstrates an injury, such as a greenstick fracture, but also reveals several other injuries of varying date, healed fractured ribs, etc. A classical site for such damage is the epiphysis of a long bone, showing on the X-ray as displacement of the epiphysis or irregularity of the epiphyseal line. A fresh epiphyseal injury may be accompanied by older injuries at several other epiphyses.

The epiphyseal injuries in particular are caused by traction on the child's limbs, not by normal childhood falls or bumps, and are produced by maltreatment by adults, deliberately or due to ignorance.

If the violence inflicted on the child continues, sooner or later severe internal injury, such as intra-cranial haemorrhage or rupture of an abdominal organ, will occur, and is likely to cause the child's death.

However, extreme care must be taken in diagnosing such a case. Severe internal injuries, particularly sub-dural haemorrhage, may be produced accidentally by falls, and surprisingly gross damage can be inflicted by other children. Solitary injuries can almost always have an accidental explanation. But if there are multiple severe injuries of varying date, if they are of a type which couldn't be produced accidentally, and especially if any of the surface injuries, e.g. bruises or abrasions, have a pattern which enables the agent to be identified, e.g. a whip or a belt, then it is almost certain that the injuries have been produced by a parent or other adult.

One should be wary of allowing apparent malnutrition or an unkempt appearance of the child to influence one's opinion on the causation of the injuries. The malnutrition may prove to be due to natural disease, and this of itself may cause the child to be more liable to fall and sustain injuries. However, if a dead child is seen who is thin, and bruised, naturally a suspicion of cruelty will be aroused, and such cases must be referred to the Coroner. A living child seen in hospital involves greater problems, since allegations of cruelty may be incorrect and cause the parents great suffering, yet the doctor has a duty to the child; if it is being maltreated and is not protected, further and fatal injuries may occur. In any case of doubt consultations should be held with the N.S.P.C.C. or the local Children's Officer, or the Health Visitor. It is unwise to notify the police at once, unless irrefutable evidence of cruelty can be produced.

Cot deaths

This name is applied to a condition of unknown aetiology, causing about 1,000 deaths each year of children between 4 and 12 months of age. It is of importance because the deaths are totally unexpected, and so may arouse suspicion of foul play, especially when they occur in families in poor social circumstances. The children usually are quite well on the day before death, or may have a cold. They are fed and put to bed in the evening, and are found dead in their cots in the morning, often lying face down. The cause of the death is not known, but the histological appearance of the lungs is reasonably characteristic, and suggestions have been put forward that the deaths are due to fulminating infection, to allergy to cow's milk proteins inhaled in minute amounts, or to inhalation of stomach contents, causing an inhalation pneumonia.

At all events, histological examination of the lungs will reveal the condition; before such examination became a routine procedure these deaths were usually ascribed to suffocation or overlaying, with the implication of negligence on the parents' part, causing quite unwarranted distress.

This is not to say that suffocation or overlaying does not occur, but a distinction should be possible if a thorough post-mortem examination is made.

Legal protection of children

A number of laws have been framed to protect children from various hazards. The principal is the Children and Young Persons Act 1933, which defines certain offences, e.g.:

Overlaying

It is an offence for a person over 16 years, when drunk, to take a child under 3 years of age into bed with him, whereby the child dies.

Protection of fires

It is an offence if a person over 16 years, who has charge of a child under 12 years, allows the child to be in a room where the fire or heating appliance is not adequately guarded.

Neglect

Any person over 16 years, having charge of a child under that age, who assaults, ill-treats, neglects, abandons, or exposes him, in a manner likely to cause unnecessary suffering or injury, commits a misdemeanour.

Non-flammable clothing

Under the Nightdresses Safety Regulations 1967, the use of any fabric in making or trimming children's nightdresses which does not conform with specified requirements of low flammability is prohibited.

However, this does not prevent parents from buying inflammable material and making up nightdresses themselves, and the doctor, by drawing the attention of parents to the dangers of such clothing, may be able to prevent severe or fatal injury to a child.

CHAPTER 21
Criminal Abortion

Legal definition

The offence of criminal abortion has been defined in the Offences Against the Person Act of 1861. To paraphrase, this states:

A woman may commit this offence, if, being pregnant, she attempts to procure her own abortion by using any instrument, poison, or other means. Another person can be guilty if he or she attempts unlawfully to procure a woman's abortion, by any means, irrespective of whether the woman 'patient' is pregnant or not. The offence is a very grave one, carrying a maximum punishment of life imprisonment, and of course if the victim dies the abortionist will be guilty of manslaughter. In the case of a doctor who procures an abortion illegally, in addition to the punishment fixed by the statute he is almost certain to be struck off the Medical Register.

Apart from the grave offence of actively procuring an abortion, it is also an offence for a person to supply an instrument, drug, or any other thing to a woman knowing that it is to be used to procure an abortion.

Lawful or unlawful abortion

It is obviously important for a doctor to know whether an abortion which he feels should be performed would be considered lawful, or unlawful. Such a decision must be based on the provisions of the Abortion Act 1967. For details see Chapter 4.

Incidence of criminal abortion

The importance of the problem of criminal abortion is indicated by the number of cases, and the risks entailed for the victims.

The actual number of criminal abortions is obviously unknown. Prior to the Abortion Act reasoned estimates put it at about 50,000 cases a year. Though probably less now, recent reports suggest that it is still far from negligible. The mortality appears to be low, probably due to the use of antibiotics, but the morbidity is high, and the potential dangers of infection, injury and death for any woman undergoing such a procedure are very great.

Methods used to procure abortion

General Violence

Attempts may be made to produce abortion by taking increased and unaccustomed physical exercise, such as gardening, horse-riding, games, etc. This is very rarely effective unless an abortion was likely to occur anyway.

More dangerous is general physical violence directly applied to the body, either by the woman, e.g. throwing herself downstairs, or by another person, e.g. the father, punching and kicking the woman's body and abdomen. While unlikely to terminate the pregnancy, such violence may inflict serious injuries on the mother such as a ruptured spleen.

Local Violence

The object of these procedures is to dilate the cervix and dislodge the ovum so that it will be expelled. This may be achieved by:

1 *Instruments.* These range from curettes or ovum forceps, used by professional abortionists, to knitting needles and hatpins by the woman herself. In skilful hands these may be very effective and safe, but used clumsily, especially by the mother herself, they are likely to produce grave injuries of the genital tract.

2 *Syringing.* A Higginson's syringe, which may be equipped with an extra long nozzle, is used to project a jet of water containing soap or disinfectant into the vagina. The nozzle may be inserted into the cervix. The object is to drive a 'fluid wedge' between the placenta and the uterine wall, with resulting expulsion of the foetus. This is probably the most commonly used method, and is reasonably effective. Its peculiar danger is the production of an embolus of air or soap which is usually immediately fatal.

3 *Slippery elm.* An uncommon method, this consists of using a sliver of wood from the bark of a tree. This wood has the property of absorbing moisture and swelling, and when inserted into the cervix, will cause dilatation, and then induce uterine contractions, in the same way as laminaria tents which have been used in obstetrics. The main hazard is the inability to sterilise the wood, and the risk of its piercing the tissues of the genital tract.

4 *Pastes.* Various pastes can be obtained, in compressible tubes, with applicators to be inserted into the cervix. The principle, similar to the syringing method, is to force a wedge beneath the placenta. This method is effective and is used by some obstetricians. Its chief hazards are of fat embolism, or of sensitivity to the constituents of the paste, notably iodine.

Abortifacient Drugs

Almost any poisonous or medicinal substance may be used by the lay person. Those commonly used are:

1   Substances supposed to increase menstrual flow. These include the typical 'old wives' remedies—purgatives such as castor oil or epsom salts; vegetable poisons like pennyroyal, tansy and apiol; 'tonics', usually compound 'female' pills containing iron and quinine among other things; and corrosives, especially potassium permanganate which, used as an intra-vaginal tablet produces ulceration and so haemorrhage, resembling an inevitable abortion, which may be treated as such by an unwary doctor.

2   Substances causing uterine contraction, ergot, pituitrin, quinine and heavy metals such as lead or mercury. Quinine is particularly dangerous as it is liable to cause permanent deafness or blindness if the victim survives.

Times of using various methods

Although, of course, not rigidly applicable, there tends to be a regular sequence of the different methods employed in early pregnancy, e.g.:

1   1st month—pregnancy uncertain—general violence.
2   2nd month—pregnancy certain—abortifacient drugs.
3   3rd month—desperation—local violence.

Dangers of abortion to the mother

General violence

Considerable violence inflicted on or by the mother may cause gross intra-abdominal or thoracic injuries, such as ruptured liver or spleen, fractured ribs or pelvis, etc., with shock and haemorrhage.

Drugs

The obvious danger is of poisoning which is likely to occur from almost any of the drugs used for this purpose, e.g. apiol may cause peripheral neuritis, pennyroyal—renal tubular necrosis, quinine—cranial nerve damage, etc.

Local violence

Immediate hazards—vagal inhibition, during dilatation of or injury to the cervix. Embolism, of air, soap or paste, during the course of syringing, or insertion of paste. Massive haemorrhage, from lacerations or penetrating wounds involving large blood vessels.

Delayed hazards (a few days)—infection, usually a fulminating clostridial septicaemia.
Haemorrhage, secondary PPH.
Renal tubular necrosis.

Late (one or more weeks)—pelvic pyaemia, chronic infections, etc.
Venous thrombosis, in pelvic or leg veins with danger of pulmonary embolism.

Circumstances in which a doctor may be involved in a criminal abortion

Doctor requested to perform an abortion by a patient

Directly. This may, of course, be a perfectly genuine case in which there prove to be adequate medical grounds for termination of pregnancy, under the provisions of the Abortion Act, 1967. If there are no adequate medical grounds abortion must be refused but every effort made, by arranging financial and other assistance for the mother, to prevent her seeking unqualified assistance, and being exposed to the dangers of criminal abortion.

By guile. Thus an unknown patient may claim that she is away from home and has a retroversion in need of correction, hoping that the examination and manipulation will cause her to abort.

The doctor is called to treat a patient who he discovers is suffering from the effects of a criminal abortion induced by another person

On occasions doctors have been criticised for not having informed the police in such circumstances. Therefore in 1916 the College of Physicians sought legal advice and formulated a code of conduct to be followed on such occasions:

(a) The doctor must never disclose the cause of his patient's condition to anyone else without the patient's consent, unless ordered to do so in Court.

(b) He should urge the patient to make a statement to the police, or, when appropriate, a dying declaration. If this is refused he should continue to treat the patient, but may seek other professional advice, medical or legal, e.g. from his medical defence society.

(c) If the patient dies then the doctor must refer the case to the Coroner as being a death due to unnatural causes.

The doctor is called to a sudden death due to abortion

The doctor is not likely to know that an abortion has been performed before he examines the body. An abortionist will obviously try to keep this secret. Therefore the doctor would be wise to treat all sudden deaths in women of childbearing age with suspicion until the cause has been established. When such a sudden death is due to abortion the mechanism will usually be either vagal inhibition or embolism of air or soap. Such a death will usually occur abruptly during the procedure, so that normally the body will be found where the abortion was being performed, at the patient's home or that of the abortionist.

If self-induced the general appearance of the body and its surroundings may indicate the circumstances, e.g. a body laid on the bed, legs apart, without pants, and with an instrument, or a syringe and bowl of soapy water nearby. However the victim may live long enough to clear away instruments, etc., and if the abortion was performed by others they will undoubtedly have removed incriminating evidence. Then the only indication may be from the clothing, such as panties worn back to front or inside out, or a small amount of foamy fluid in the vagina, possibly smelling of disinfectant.

In such cases, as in any type of 'criminal' death, the doctor must remember to be very careful not to touch anything except the body at the scene. Vital fingerprints on instruments, bowls, glasses, etc., may otherwise be lost.

Autopsy

Although known cases of abortion will usually be the responsibility of a forensic pathologist, an unsuspected case may turn up in ordinary autopsy work.

The possibility should always be considered at any autopsy on the body of a woman of childbearing age. It is wise, in such a case, to open the abdomen first and inspect the uterus. If this is enlarged, as by pregnancy, then a careful examination must be made for signs of uterine or vaginal injury, air embolism, etc.

It is important to retain samples of right heart blood and vaginal or intra-uterine fluid for analysis for any disinfectants, etc., which may be present.

CHAPTER 22
Infanticide

At and shortly after birth a child is liable to succumb to one or other of many natural diseases. However, it is equally vulnerable to injury and whenever the dead body of a newly-born infant is seen, especially if the body had been concealed, the possibility that the child had been deliberately killed must be considered. Such a killing might be murder, but under certain circumstances if done by the mother the crime will be that of infanticide.

Infanticide—the law

The distinction of this crime, by Act of Parliament in 1938 (the Infanticide Act), was due to an appreciation that a woman might, because of birth or lactation, be suffering from mental disturbance and so be only partly responsible for her actions—a forerunner (in England) of the doctrine of diminished responsibility.

To paraphrase the law, when a woman kills her child, provided that the child is less than one year old, and provided that it can be shown that at the time the woman's mental state was disturbed by the after-effects of delivery, or the effects of lactation, then the crime will not be murder, but will be infanticide. This crime is equivalent to manslaughter and is usually dealt with by putting the mother on probation.

Circumstances involving the doctor

When any child less than one year old dies it may be the

victim of infanticide, but the question usually arises when the circumstances are suspicious, e.g.:

1 When a woman is found with a newly-delivered dead child, especially if the child is unwanted or illegitimate, and there were no witnesses of the birth.

2 When the dead body of a newly-born baby is found abandoned or concealed, with no indication of the identity of the mother.

Examination of the child

When the doctor is called upon to examine the body it is useful for him to have a scheme by which to work. This should cover three points:

1 Was the child viable?

2 Did the child have a separate existence, or was it still-born?

3 What was the cause of death, or still-birth?

Viability

This is a legal concept, not to be confused with medical terms indicating a living state, e.g. viable tissue.

It is an estimate of the unborn child's chance of survival, should it be delivered at any stage prior to full-term. The period of gestation of 28 weeks is the arbitrary point chosen. A foetus of less than 28 weeks' gestation is considered to have almost no chance of survival if born, and is called non-viable, whereas a foetus of more than 28 weeks is viable, i.e. if born it is likely to survive.

The distinction is important in law, e.g. in the crime of Child Destruction (see below), and provides the layman with a yardstick with which to assess the evidence of a live birth in a charge of infanticide.

The maturity of a child can be assessed:

Externally. 1 From the general appearance, size, and development.

2   From the weight—viable infants weigh over $2\frac{1}{2}$ lb.

3   From the length. This is the most convenient method.

The measurement is from the crown of the head to the heel. For the first 5 months of gestation the length in cm is the square of the age, e.g. 3 months 9 cm, 4 months 16 cm. After 5 months the length in cm divided by 5, or in inches divided by 2 is the age in months, e.g.:

$14/2$ in $= 7$ months (28 weeks) $= 35/5$ cm.

Internally. At autopsy additional evidence of maturity can be obtained:

1   From the skeletal development, i.e. the occurrence of centres of ossification. These are not precise indices, but centres are likely to be present in the foot, in the talus and calcaneum at 28 weeks, at the lower end of the femur after 36 weeks, and the upper end of the tibia after 40 weeks. They can be found by direct inspection on cutting across the bone ends with a knife, or by X-ray.

2   From dental data. X-ray or dissection will show the stage of development and calcification of the teeth, and maturity can be judged from this by a dentist who is experienced in this procedure.

Separate Existence

A child cannot be considered live-born unless it has shown signs of life when completely separated from the mother. This means that the whole of its body is separated, i.e. a child that is breathing when the head is delivered, but dies while one foot is still in the vagina, is in fact a still-birth. The placenta and umbilical cord do not however count as part of the body, i.e. a living child whose body is completely extruded is a live birth, even though still attached by the umbilical cord to a placenta in the uterus.

Signs of life are defined for purposes of registration under the Births and Deaths Registration Act 1953 as breathing, beating of the heart, pulsation of the umbilical cord or definite movement of voluntary muscles.

Therefore when examining a baby's body it is necessary to show that the breathing, heart beat or movement had occurred when the child had achieved separation from the mother. It is obvious that this is always difficult, and frequently impossible, to prove.

(a) *Signs on external examination*

Of live birth	*Of still-birth*
Separation of the umbilical cord.	Maceration—this only occurs in intra-uterine death.
Drying and shrivelling occurs in about 24 hours, separation in 4–5 days after birth.	Conditions incompatible with life, e.g. gross malformation, head in a caul.

(b) *Signs on internal examination*

Of live birth	*Of still-birth*
Lungs obviously fully expanded by breathing in a recently dead baby.	Gross congenital abnormalities, incompatible with life, e.g. certain forms of congenital heart disease.

Lungs which are partially or unexpanded must be examined microscopically with the minimum of handling prior to fixation. Evidence of live birth may then be given by the presence of hyaline membrane or pulmonary oedema, and of still-birth by findings of flooding of the lungs by amniotic fluid with squames and meconium in the alveolae, or early maceration with desquamation of bronchial epithelium. Bronchopneumonia may occur in still- or live-born infants.

Remember. Partial expansion of the lungs by breathing is not *proof* of separate existence; a period of breathing may occur with the child only partially delivered, if at an unattended delivery the mother collapses from pain or shock.

Putrefaction will destroy all but the most obvious signs of live birth, i.e. separation of the cord and food in the stomach. In the absence of these, the infant must be assumed to be stillborn, since the contrary cannot be proved, and so the mother should be given the benefit of any doubt.

Cause of death

Once the facts of viability and separate existence have been considered the third point, of cause of death, must be decided.

Common Causes of Still-birth

Prematurity.
Congenital abnormalities, notably of the CVS and CNS.
Birth trauma—such as brain damage.
Anoxia—as from prolapsed cord.
Placental insufficiency.
Infection—intra-uterine pneumonia.
Blood disorders—erythroblastosis foetalis.

Common Causes of Natural Neonatal Death

Any of the above conditions may cause death after a period of extra-uterine existence. In addition:
Respiratory distress syndrome—hyaline membrane disease.
Cranial birth trauma—meningeal tears and intra-cranial haemorrhage.
Infections, bronchopneumonia, umbilical sepsis with septi-caemia, etc.
Massive pulmonary haemorrhage.
None of the conditions in these first two groups are likely to show signs by which they can be diagnosed externally.

Causes of unnatural death

(a) *Acts of omission.* (These are usually involuntary, due to illness or ignorance of the mother at an unattended delivery.)

Obstruction of the airways by amniotic fluid—failure to suck out and position the child.

Drowning—precipitate delivery in a toilet.

Hypothermia—exposure after delivery, in cold weather, when no provision has been made for the birth.

Strangulation by the cord—failure to relieve the pressure during delivery.

(b) *Acts of commission.* These are deliberate acts designed to cause the child's death:

Common. (a) *Suffocation.* By obstruction of the nostrils and mouth by bedding, or by the mother's fingers.

(b) *Head injuries.* By hitting the head with an object, such as a fist, or by swinging the body by the feet so as to dash the head against the wall.

Remember that fractures of the skull, cracks extending laterally from the sagittal suture, and intra-cranial bleeding, may occur naturally during birth. However, following deliberate injury the injuries reflect the greater violence. There is likely to be damage, abrasion or laceration of the scalp, the fractures will be larger and probably multiple, usually with laceration of the underlying dura and laceration of the brain.

(c) *Strangulation.* This may be by the hands, with bruising and nail scratches. Similar marks may be produced by the hands during self-delivery, but are then probably distributed widely over the surface of the head, on the eyebrows, ears and the chest. Alternatively a ligature may be used, such as a piece of string. The umbilical cord may be used as the ligature and will then probably be bruised and torn by the rough handling distinguishing the circumstances from accidental strangulation by the cord during delivery. In all the circumstances the head in a recently dead baby will be congested with petechial haemorrhages on the skin and face, and there is likely to be bruising of the neck structures at autopsy.

Less Common. (a) *Stabbing*—often by some convenient agent such as (nail) scissors used to cut the cord. If a single wound it may be suggested that this occurred accidentally whilst the cord was being cut. Alternatively a sharp object such as a knitting needle may be thrust into the fontanelle, or the eye.

(b) *Cut throat*—by scissors, a knife or a razor blade. They are often ragged with multiple wounds due to the panic of the mother.

(c) *Drowning*—by holding the child's face in a bowl or bucket of fluid. It may be possible to prove this by finding material, such as soap, in the fluid in the lungs, otherwise it is usually impossible to distinguish from accidental drowning due to precipitate delivery. Immersion is a common mode of disposal of the body after infanticide by other means, or after stillbirth.

Rare. Burning; Poisoning; Burial alive, etc.

All the unnatural causes of death will probably leave visible external signs, but while these may excite suspicion, it would be unwise to make a definite diagnosis without autopsy examination.

Child destruction

This crime was defined in order to bridge a gap in the law which existed between abortion and infanticide, and is set out in the Infant Life Preservation Act 1929.

The Act makes it an offence to cause the death of a child which is unborn but viable, i.e. of 28 weeks' gestation or more while *in utero*.

However, medical procedures, such as craniotomy, done to preserve the mother's life, are excluded.

Child destruction is difficult to prove, even after autopsy examination, and few are charged with this grave offence.

Concealment of birth

The law, in the Offence Against the Person Act, 1861, makes it an offence to hide a newly-born child's body so as to conceal the fact of birth. It is immaterial whether the child is viable or not, whether it was live or stillborn, or how it died. It is not even necessary to have discovered the child's body, if the mother can be proved to have been recently delivered. Concealment must be proved, but the criteria of this are legal, not medical matters.

It is a crime which does not carry a serious punishment, and is often charged as an alternative to infanticide. Upon conviction the woman is usually bound over, or put on probation.

CHAPTER 23
Identification

Identification of the living

This problem may arise in hospital when an unknown person is brought in unconscious, or when a conscious person suffers from amnesia, e.g. following a head injury. The determination of the identity of the unknown person is ultimately the responsibility of the police, but the doctor may be required to assist, by providing a detailed physical description. The main points to consider are listed below.

General appearance

e.g. height, weight, sex, approximate age, colouring of skin, hair, and eyes.

Clothing

This is usually dealt with by the police, who list the clothing, examine it for laundry or other marks, and search the pockets for identifying papers, tickets, etc. Similarly all cash and jewellery must be recorded.

Fingerprints

This also is a police responsibility. The prints, of the skin ridges from the fingers, and sometimes from the palms, are taken by ink impressions on paper. The basic types of fingerprint shape are arches, loops and whorls, but the patterns are so complex that no two prints from different people have ever been found to be the same, and even identical twins can be distinguished. The object of taking fingerprints from an unidentified person is so that the police can compare the prints with those on their files, of known persons, or when a possible identity has been suggested, can compare the unknown person's prints with prints on objects known to have been used by that person.

Fingerprint patterns are unaltered by age, or injury, so that prints made years earlier can safely be used for comparison.

Scars

These do not have the unique quality of fingerprints, for instance there must be many people alive with appendicectomy scars, but scars may be of use in distinguishing between two possible identities if only one person is known to have such a scar. Of course the greater number of scars present and the more unusual their character the more useful they will be in proving identity. Their site, exact shape and size, and approximate age must be recorded.

It should be remembered that small scars may become undetectable with age, especially linear scars from incised wounds.

Tattoos

As with scars, these are not unique, but may be very useful distinguishing features. The more elaborate and colourful the design the better, though colours fade with time, especially green and red.

Mentality

In a conscious, amnesic patient, an assessment of his mental ability and education may be of value.

Anthropometry

On the Continent systems of identification, notably the Bertillon system, have been designed which use photographs and complex measurements, especially of head shape.

The best known medico-legal cases of identification of the living have usually involved the detection of impostors claiming estates, or the establishment of the identity of a person wrongly accused of a crime. However, such cases are rare and are very unlikely to be within the province of most doctors.

Identification of the dead

This provides one of the most fascinating aspects of forensic

pathology. The problem usually arises in one of three forms:
1   A recently dead and unmutilated corpse is discovered, e.g. in a river, but with no means of identification from documents, licences, etc.
2   A body or group of bodies is gravely injured, e.g. in an aircraft crash or a fire, so that visual identification is impossible, but the size, sex, and approximate age are obvious.
3   Some grossly decomposed or skeletal human remains are discovered. The size, sex and age of the deceased cannot be determined by simple inspection of the remains.

The procedure to be adopted will obviously vary in each type of case.

Recently dead and undamaged body

When dealing with such a body it should be possible to produce a detailed description of the external appearance of the deceased, as in the case of a living person, and combine with this any evidence of natural disease, or previous injuries or operations revealed at autopsy.

Recently dead but badly damaged body

In such a case the sex, height, and approximate age of the deceased are usually readily determined by simple inspection of the body. However, the impossibility of facial recognition makes it necessary to search for other distinguishing features. These may be found in the remnants of clothing, jewellery, etc., which are present on the body, or there may be distinctive scars, tattoos or physical deformities. However, the most reliable evidence is likely to be obtained from dental investigation. An accurate dental chart should be compiled by a dentist, and may then be compared with the dental records of the various people known, for instance, to have been in the aircraft, if, as is nowadays more commonly the case, the problem of identification arises in relation to the victims of an air crash.

Alternatively, dentures may be identified by the dentist who made them, and in some countries it is nowadays the practice to insert identifying tags into the material of the denture.

Skeletal remains

It is first necessary to decide whether the remains are of human origin, or the bones of some animal, and also how many individuals are represented.

If human, the problem then is to establish the primary characteristics of the deceased, i.e. sex, age, and height. Having thereby produced a bare outline of a person, the next object is to fill into this outline as many other details as possible by which the remains can be identified.

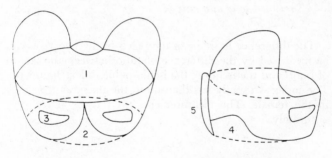

Fig. 13. *Female pelvis. 1. General pelvic shape— flat bowl; 2. Sub-pubic arch—obtuse; 3. Obturator foramen—oval; 4. Sciatic notch—obtuse; 5. Sacrum—short and flat.*

Primary characteristics. 1. Sex—In adults fortunately there are well-marked differences between the bones of the two sexes after puberty. The most useful parts of the skeleton in this respect are the pelvis, and the skull.

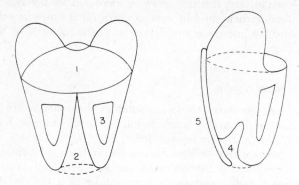

FIG. 14. *Male pelvis. 1. General pelvic shape—deep funnel; 2. Sub-pelvic arch—acute; 3. Obturator foramen—triangular; 4. Sciatic notch—acute; 5. Sacrum—long and curved.*

The difference in shape of the pelvis in the two sexes can be measured by the difference of ratio between the length of pubis and the ischium, the ischio-pubic index (figure 15). The index is usually less than 90 in the male, and over 90 in the female. The measurements need to be made very accurately.

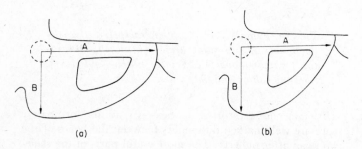

FIG. 15. *(See text.) (a) Female, (b) male.*

In the case of a female, there is a well-marked groove on the front of the ilium close to its attachment to the sacrum, called the pre-auricular groove, and produced by the attachment of a ligament.

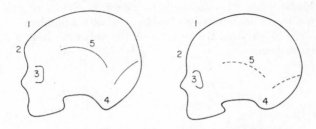

FIG. 16. *Male skull. 1. Forehead—receding; 2. Orbital ridges—prominent; 3. Orbits—square; 4. Mastoid process—large; 5. Muscle ridges—marked.*

FIG. 17. *Female skull. 1. Forehead—high; 2. Orbital ridges—not marked; 3. Orbits—rounded; 4. Mastoid process—small; 5. Muscle ridges—faint.*

Long bones—In the male the bones are more massive, especially the articular regions, and the ridges for muscle attachment are more prominent.

Soft tissue—If the remains are only partially decomposed and not reduced to a skeleton, it may be possible from examination of soft tissue to determine the sex microscopically, by detection of the sex chromatin masses in the cell nuclei, mainly in skin or cartilage. However, this is rarely possible, due to putrefactive changes. The main value of this method is in the examination of a small part of a recently dismembered body.

2. *Age* (a) *From the bones.* From soon after conception to early adult life age is assessed from the development of

ossific centres, and the fusion of these to the ends of the bones. Although the times of appearance of the ossific centres and union of epiphyses are not absolutely constant, the maximum range of variation is only of the order of 1–2 years, and therefore a reasonably reliable estimate of age can be made. It is advisable to consult textbooks or practitioners of anatomy when dealing with such a problem.

Up to 30 years the surfaces of the vertebrae bear well-marked furrows.

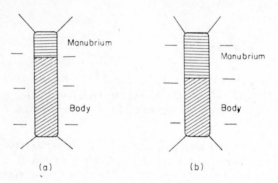

FIG. 18. *Sternum: (a) male, (b) female.*

After 30 years age can only be approximately assessed, by the closure of skull sutures, and the onset of degenerative changes, such as osteoarthritis. Again textbooks of anatomy should be consulted for the approximate times and the variations in the closure of the skull sutures.

(b) *From the teeth* (such work obviously should be carried out by a dentist).

Before birth—specialised techniques exist for determining the extent of development of the teeth in the jaws, by dissection and possibly by determination of the mineral content.

In childhood—the state of eruption of the teeth of the primary or secondary dentition on direct inspection, possibly coupled with X-ray of the jaws to determine the extent of calcification of the unerupted teeth, gives a reliable indication of age, up to late adolescence.

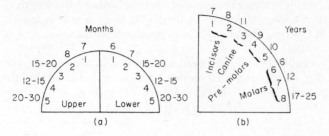

FIG. 19. (a) *Primary dentition*, (b) *secondary dentition*.

In adults—the extent of wear of the teeth, as assessed by an experienced dentist, on ground sections, may give some indication of age. The method was developed first in Scandinavia by Gustafson.

Such a method can only be applied with any degree of reliability by a dentist, who has experience of its application, and even then his estimate is no more than approximate.

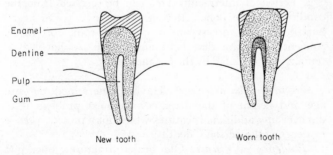

FIG. 20

3. Height—The determination of this depends on the principle that there is a fixed relationship between the length of the limbs, especially the legs, and the total length of the body. Therefore if the length of a long bone from a limb is accurately measured and the ratio of the length of this bone, e.g. femur, to the whole body length is known, the person's height can be determined, with an accuracy of $\pm$ 1 in.

Tables of ratios between the length of a whole body, and the component long bones have been prepared by the examination of large numbers of cadavers—e.g. from Dupertius and Hadden's tables (for dry bones without cartilage):

(a) *Male:*

Length femur $\times$ 2·238 + 69·089 cm or 27·200 in.
Length tibia $\times$ 2·392 + 81·688 cm or 32·161 in.

(b) *Female:*

Length femur $\times$ 2·317 + 61·412 cm or 24·178 in.
Length tibia $\times$ 2·533 + 72·572 cm or 28·572 in.

Similar formulae are available for other bones, such as the humerus and radius, and for combinations of measurements of different bones. The measurements must be made precisely, using an osteometric board, not tape-measures, etc.

4. Period of interment—This can be assessed from the condition of the bones. Recent bones (e.g. 10–20 years' burial) are firm, greasy and may retain some soft tissue. Ancient bones are dry, light and brittle. Archaeological remains can be dated by the C_{14} method.

Secondary characteristics. Having determined the sex, age and height of the deceased, the next problem is to discover any additional features which may provide precise evidence of the person's identity.

1 *Evidence of disease.* Old healed fractures, operation scars on the skull, arthritis, etc. X-rays of the skeleton may

be valuable. In addition, in the partially decomposed body gall-stones or uterine fibroids may be detected.

2 *Dental evidence.* Often skulls may lose teeth during putrefaction, and disinterment, or may be edentate. However, where teeth are present, an accurate record of their position, condition and any fillings, etc., should be made, preferably by a dentist. These records can then be compared with the dental records of missing persons.

PART THREE

Toxicology

It is generally agreed that there is no simple classification into which all the important poisons can be fitted. This is unfortunate for the student, but the only attempt made here to classify poisons is by their principal symptom.

CHAPTER 24

Poisoning—Diagnosis and Treatment

Diagnosis

The decision that a person's illness is due to poison can be an extremely difficult one to make. One reason for this may be lack of suspicion in the doctor's mind, so that the possibility of poison is not even considered.

Also the signs and symptoms produced by poisons are so varied, and may mimic natural disease so closely that there may be nothing in the patient's condition which is distinctive of poison.

Fortunately the history often indicates that poison is responsible for the illness, and the nature of the poison may be known, or the tablets or liquids which have been consumed may be brought to the doctor. Otherwise, the circumstances in which poison should automatically be considered at the outset of a possible cause of the illness are:

1 Sudden onset of severe illness in children.

2 Sudden illness in a person known to have been previously completely healthy, especially the sudden onset of coma.

3 Sudden illness or coma in a person suffering from depression or any mental disturbance.

4 Illness in a man whose work brings him into contact with poisonous substances, i.e. most industrial and agricultural occupations.

Even then, cases of poisoning will occur where the circumstances give no grounds for suspicion, e.g. cases of accidental domestic poisoning and unexpected suicides, especially among persons already suffering from severe natural disease.

Some poisons have effects which make their presence obvious, e.g. burning of the mouth by corrosives, pink coloration of the skin in carbon monoxide poisoning or grey-brown due to methaemoglobin, but many poisons do not have characteristic features and present symptoms of a general nature.

Therefore, the doctor should endeavour to include the appropriate poisons in the differential diagnosis of each major symptom, as suggested below.

This list is not intended to be exhaustive, but to act as a guide. Students could benefit by preparing more detailed lists of their own.

Acute gastro-intestinal disorder

e.g. vomiting, diarrhoea and abdominal pain

Disease	*Poison*
Infective gastro-enteritis	Corrosives, acids,
'Acute abdomen'	alkalis, etc.
Cerebral disorders,	Irritant metals
acute infections in	and metalloids
childhood	

Chronic alimentary disorders

e.g. abdominal pain, constipation or diarrhoea, loss of weight and anoxexia, etc.

Disease	*Poison*
Neoplasm	Metals, notably lead
Ulcerative colitis	and arsenic
Steatorrhoea	
Chronic infections	

Delirium

Disease	Poison
Cerebral disease-infection or haemorrhage, or tumour	Alcohols
	Antifreeze
	Bromides
Anoxic—from haemorrhage or cardio-vascular or respiratory disease	Amphetamine
	Atropine
	Cocaine, cannabis
	Lead (tetraethyl)
Pyrexia—especially in the elderly	Barbiturates
Metabolic disorders such as uraemia, and vitamin B deficiency	

Coma

Disease	Poison
Cerebro-vascular accidents	Barbiturates
Head injury, electric shock	Aspirin
Myxoedema, metabolic causes, e.g. diabetes, psychoses, hypothermia	Carbon monoxide
	Narcotics
	Insulin
	Alcohol
	Cyanide
	Phenol
	Tranquillisers
	Chloral
	Paraldehyde

Convulsions with or without coma

Disease	Poison
Epilepsy, encephalitis	Strychnine, lead
Tetanus, hysteria	Camphor

Cerebro-vascular accidents   Cocaine, atropine
Quinine, amphetamine
Laburnam

Acute paralysis or peripheral neuritis

Disease	Poison
Poliomyelitis	Alcohol, meths
Encephalitis	Lead arsenic
Cerebro-vascular disorders	Thallium, mercury
Diabetic neuritis	T.O.C.P., parathion
Motor neurone diseases	Quinine
Disseminated sclerosis	Nicotine, cyanide
Polyarteritis	Aconite
Porphyria	Hemlock

Alternatively, if poisoning is suspected, the likely poisons available in the particular circumstances can be considered, e.g.:

Common suicidal poisons

Carbon monoxide, barbiturates, aspirin, tranquillisers.

Common household poisons

Corrosives, phenols, bleach, methyl alcohol, petrol, paraffin, creosote, polishes (containing aniline or nitrobenzene, etc.), stain removers (containing oxalate), hair perms (containing pot. bromate), rat poisons (barium or dicoumarol), dry-cleaning agents (containing carbon tetrachloride), etc.

Common medicinal poisons

At home—barbiturates, tranquillisers, bromides, strychnine, digitalis, narcotics, iron preparations, antihistamines.
     Anaesthetic agents in hospital.

Common industrial poisons

Gases—CO, N_2O, SO_2, $COCl_4$, H_2S, SO_2, CS_2.

Metals—lead, mercury, arsenic, antimony, chrome, beryllium, cadmium, cyanide.

Metalloids—phosphorus, and organic phosphates, fluorides.

Organic—halogenated hydrocarbons—e.g. carbon tetrachloride, trichlorethane, methyl chloride and bromide, etc.

Common poisons in childhood

Aspirin, tranquillisers, iron preparations, barbiturates, antihistamines, strychnine, borates, lead, poisonous plants, berries, and mushrooms.

Treatment

Once poison is suspected from the clinical signs and symptoms, chemical tests must be made to determine its exact nature. This may be a protracted procedure, and in the case of acute poisoning treatment must usually be instituted before the nature of the poison is known for certain. Fortunately, the main lines of treatment are independent of the nature of the poison.

The treatment of any poisoning is basically directed by three principles:

1 Separate the patient from the poison.
2 Keep the patient alive—symptomatic treatment.
3 Give specific treatment, i.e. antidotes, where applicable.

The order in which one carries out these three lines of treatment depends on the circumstances of the individual case, and is dictated by common sense. Thus symptomatic treatment for a gaseous poison is useless while the victim remains in the contaminated atmosphere, and equally, meticulous washing out of the stomach for an ingested

poison is of no avail if the patient dies of respiratory failure
during the procedure.

Separating the patient from the poison. The method
adopted depends on the route by which the poison has been
absorbed, i.e.:

(a) *Inhaled gaseous poisons*—remove the patient from the
contaminated atmosphere, and administer oxygen, with
artificial respiration, if necessary.

(b) *Ingested poisons*—if seen soon after the poison has
been swallowed, provided that it is not a corrosive, vomiting may be produced (emesis) by putting a finger down
the throat, or by salt water (1 dessertspoon per tumbler of
water) or mustard (1 teaspoon per tumbler of water).

As soon as admitted to hospital, if the general condition
is satisfactory, the stomach should be washed out, using a
stomach tube (not a Ryle's tube), through which small
quantities—1 to 2 pints—of tepid water are alternately
poured into and syphoned out of the stomach. The tech-
nique can only be learnt practically in the Casualty Department, but one main precaution is to protect the airway, by
seeing that the tube is not passed into the trachea, and,
in an unconscious patient, by passing a cuffed endotracheal
tube and positioning the patient so that the mouth is at a
lower level than the lungs.

(c) *Skin contamination*—contaminated clothing must be
removed and the skin gently but adequately washed, with
large amounts of warm water. No scrubbing, as this will
increase absorption.

(d) *Injected poisons*—if injected subcutaneously the
application of ice or a tourniquet may reduce the rate of
absorption. Intra-muscular or intravenous injections are too
rapidly absorbed to make such measures practicable.

Keeping the patient alive. This simply means treatment
to counteract the various symptoms of the poisoning which
are threatening life.

(a) *Respiratory failure.* This may be merely a matter of clearing the airway in an unconscious patient, as by pulling the tongue forward, or manual artificial respiration or a mechanical respirator may be necessary.

(b) *Circulatory failure and shock.* This is along the standard lines, i.e. warmth, removal of pain by morphia, and adequate fluid intake, intravenous if necessary, with drugs to maintain blood pressure if required.

(c) *Convulsions.* Rapid sedation by intravenous barbiturates, intra-muscular paraldehyde, etc., coupled with skilled nursing designed to reduce external stimulation to a minimum.

(d) *Coma.* Treatment resides principally in nursing care, especially measures to prevent infection. Antibiotics may be required and a careful check of fluid balance to prevent dehydration, with biochemical control where necessary.

Specific treatment. Specific antidotes are few in number and are probably the least important of the methods of treatment. The effective antidotes are listed here, and details can be found under the appropriate poison.

Acid corrosives—dilute alkali (magnesia)
Alkaline corrosives—dilute acid (vinegar)
Narcotics—nalorphin or levallorphan
Arsenic and mercury—B.A.L. (dimercaprol)
Lead—E.D.T.A.
Copper—N-penicillamine
Iron—desferrioxamine
Cyanide—sodium nitrite and sodium thiosulphate: Co. E.D.T.A.
Parathion—atropine and pralidoxime
Amphetamine—chlorpromazine
Summary—shown in figure 21.

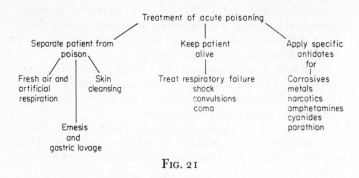

Fig. 21

Factors affecting action of poison

A knowledge of the relevant factors in any case of poisoning will aid the doctor in judging which methods of treatment are suitable, and in assessing the prognosis.

Route of absorption. Thus food in the stomach may delay the action of ingested poisons. The lethal dose of a poison by injection is usually a quarter of the oral dose, and per rectum is twice the oral dose.

Idiosyncrasy. In a person who is sensitive a much smaller dose than normal may prove fatal, e.g. in aspirin poisoning.

Age. Generally children and the aged are more susceptible to poisons, but children can tolerate relatively more atropine than adults.

Habit. A person accustomed to taking a drug may become tolerant, and may be able to take far more than the usual lethal dose.

Health. Any ill-health is likely to accelerate the effects of the poison, though on occasion local disease, e.g. chronic gastritis, may reduce its effects.

Concentration of the poison. Thus corrosives, if dilute, have little effect, however much is taken, unlike pharmacologically active substances.

Chemical form. Closely similar chemical substances may differ greatly in poisonous effects, e.g. mercuric and mercurous chlorides.

Physical states. Gases and liquids are absorbed more rapidly than powders, tablets, etc.

Dealing with a suspected case of homicidal poisoning

When a doctor suspects that one of his patients is suffering from chronic poisoning, the poison being administered by another, he has a duty to protect the life of his patient, but he would be wise to refrain from voicing his suspicions until they can be confirmed.

Such confirmation can be obtained by submitting samples, e.g. blood, urine, faeces, or hair, for analysis, using some pretext to explain the procedure to the patient. However, it is simpler to send the patient to hospital, explaining one's suspicions to the physician. During the period in hospital the patient should be safe from further administration of poison, and full investigations, including analyses, can be carried out.

If the presence of poison is confirmed, the doctor would be well advised to confer with experienced colleagues, and with his medical protection society, before informing the patient and the authorities, but obviously his guiding principle must be the welfare of his patient.

If the patient dies and poisoning is suspected to be the cause of death, then the doctor's task is relatively simple, since he must refer the case to the Coroner. However, the possibility of poison should cross the doctor's mind when dealing with any sudden death. The clues may be obvious, e.g. a cup containing powder on the bedside locker, capsules in the bed, fragments of capsule or powder on the lips or in the mouth, an unusual coloration of the post-mortem staining, etc. Also the doctor should be sure that he has a record of amounts and types of drugs which he prescribed for the patient, and should see if all the drugs can be accounted for. Often the diagnosis is only made at autopsy, since it is not uncommon for there to be no external signs to suggest poisoning, and so the doctor should be quite sure that he knows the cause of death of any of his patients who die suddenly before issuing a death certificate instead of referring the case to the Coroner.

CHAPTER 25
Common Suicidal Poisons

Barbiturates

At the present time these drugs are most commonly responsible for fatal poisoning, having succeeded carbon monoxide which previously held that distinction; with the increasing frequency of poisoning by tranquillisers and antidepressants, it seems possible that these, in turn, may succeed barbiturates as the commonest agents of fatal poisoning in the near future.

The barbiturates are in Part I of the Poisons List; they are controlled by Schedules 1 and 4a of the Poisons Regulations. They are CNS depressants and are used principally as hypnotics. There are many different varieties having different durations of action, e.g.

Long action—12–24 hours—phenobarbitone

Medium action—6–8 hours—amylobarbitone

Short action—2–4 hours—quinalbarbitone

Ultra short acting drugs, e.g. thiopentone, are used as anaesthetic agents. Therapeutic doses are usually about 15 mg for long-acting and 150 mg–200 mg for short-acting drugs.

Excretion is via the kidney in the case of the long-acting barbiturates; short acting ones are detoxified in the liver.

Lethal Dose. This is of the order of 1.5 to 2.0 G of the 15 mg for long-acting and 150 mg–200 mg for short-acting drugs.

Effects. Normal doses produce drowsiness, ataxia, and sleep. Overdoses produce an exaggeration of this, deep coma with absent reflexes, respiratory depression, peripheral circulatory failure or 'shock', loss of intestinal motility, and oliguria.

The long-acting drugs, e.g. phenobarbitone, produce a coma which may last several days. The blood level is likely to be over 8 mg per 100 ml. The danger is chiefly of infection, such as bronchopneumonia.

Short-acting drugs, e.g. seconal, produce coma lasting for about 24 hours, with blood levels above 3 mg per 100 ml. The principal dangers here are of severe respiratory depression or pulmonary oedema, of rapid onset. Death may occur within half an hour of consuming the drug, and may be associated with relatively low blood levels of the drug, as CO_2 retention and anoxia due to partial obstruction of the airway by the tongue will contribute to the cerebral depression.

Additive effects of other drugs. Any depressant drugs taken at the same time will add their effects to those of the barbiturates. This is particularly important in the case of alcohol, especially regarding driving. Small amounts of barbiturates, and of alcohol taken together, will have the depressant effects of marked intoxication and may produce sufficient respiratory depression to prove fatal. Thus in the presence of alcohol 0.6–1.0 G of amylobarbitone may prove fatal.

Laboratory Tests. In a suspected poisoning, analysis of gastric washings and of blood will show the type and amount of barbiturate in the body and indicate the mode of treatment which is required.

Treatment. This is principally symptomatic, preventing respiratory depression, circulatory failure, infection, etc. If the drug has been taken within the previous 4 hours, some may remain in the stomach and can be removed by lavage. Analeptics are only indicated in deep coma, pending removal to hospital and the institution of adequate symptomatic treatment. In very prolonged coma with high blood levels, haemodialysis may be necessary to reduce the amount of drug circulating, and so shorten the duration of coma.

Autopsy findings. Tablets or powder residues may be found at the scene of death. There are rarely any external signs on the body, but occasionally there may be large blisters on the insides of legs and arms, when coma has been prolonged.

Internally, sodium salts of barbiturates, e.g. sodium amytal, being alkaline, may produce mild corrosion of the stomach. Otherwise the signs will only be of acute heart failure.

Methaqualone

Usually taken in the form of Mandrax tablets. This drug is a strong hypnotic. In poisoning, apart from coma, there may be bizarre neurological signs, with increased reflexes and clonus or convulsions. The myocardium may be damaged, and pulmonary oedema occur. Haemorrhagic tendencies may be pronounced, especially, in fatal cases, where the appearance of the body after death may lead to a misconception that death was due to haematemesis from a peptic ulcer. Levels of drug in the blood greater than 3 mg per 100 ml may result in death, but the finding of higher levels is associated with its increasing use as a drug of addiction.

Tranquillisers

The majority of these are phenothiazine derivatives, together with a few chemically unrelated drugs, e.g. meprobamate, which are known as minor tranquillisers. These drugs are used in the treatment of psychoses and psychoneuroses. There are many of them, among the better known being chlorpromazine (Largactil), perphenazine (Fentazin), chlordiazepoxide (Librum) and trifluoperazine (Stelazine). Normal doses may produce side-effects, such as hyperactivity of the muscles of the head and neck, or a condition resembling Parkinson's disease. If the drug is given to a person suffering from coronary disease, postural hypotension may occur, with fatal results. Other serious side-effects may be various blood disorders such as thrombocytopenic purpura or haemolytic anaemia. Liver damage and jaundice may develop, and microscopic examination reveal stasis of bile in liver cell canaliculi.

Poisoning by a large overdose may produce convulsions, succeeded by coma, with hypotension and hypothermia. Treatment should be symptomatic, but avoiding analeptics and adrenaline, which may exaggerate the effect of the poison.

A few cases of unexpected sudden death of patients treated with these drugs have been reported, apparently due to abrupt heart failure. Microscopical examination has shown localised degeneration of the myocardium.

These drugs may potentiate the effects of alcohol.

Antidepressants

Some of the drugs in this group are known as mono-amine

oxidase inhibitors, since they inhibit the action of the mono-amine oxidase enzymes. An example of such a drug is phenelzine (Nardil). They act as cerebral stimulants, by allowing such substances as serotonin and nor-adrenaline to accumulate in the brain.

Another group of drugs have a cerebral depressant action, examples being imipramine and amitryptaline.

The mono-amine oxidase inhibitors are dangerous if given in combination with certain other drugs, notably pethidine, morphine, adrenaline drugs, antihistamines, cocaine, and other antidepressant drugs. Such combinations may result in violent hypertensive crises, or sudden collapse. An acute hypertensive episode may also result if cheese, which contains tyramine, is eaten while one of these drugs is being taken. It has been suggested that phentolamine mesylate or pentolinium should be used in the treatment of such hypertensive crises.

Coma may occur with overdoses of 1 G or more of the antidepressant drugs such as amitryptaline and death may result from respiratory depression. Jaundice from liver damage may occur, and the condition may, rarely, progress to total necrosis of the liver.

Overdoses of 1 G or more of the antidepressant drugs such as amitryptaline may cause coma, together with features suggesting atropine poisoning, due to the anti-cholinergic action, such as dry mouth, cardiac arrhythmias, hallucinations or convulsions, and suppression of urine; death may result from respiratory depression. Treatment may need to be especially directed towards controlling cardiac arrhythmies, with pyridostigmine or artificial pacemakers.

Salicylates

Source. Poisoning is usually by the readily available aspirin tablet, though it may also be caused by sodium salicylate, or by methyl salicylate liniment. There are no restrictions on the sale of these substances.

Lethal dose. Probably about 5–12 G of aspirin (20–50 tablets) or 5–6 ml of liniment.

Effects. Sodium salicylate readily dissolves but aspirin is less soluble and so large amounts of powder remain in the stomach for a long time. The salicylate has an irritant effect on the stomach, causing vomiting soon after ingestion of the poison, whereby much may be returned. Within a few hours the salicylate, by stimulation of the brain, causes overbreathing, acidotic in character, sweating, and coma. The overbreathing causes disturbance of the acid-base balance of the blood, producing first respiratory alkalosis, by removing CO_2, followed by compensatory metabolic acidosis. It is usually the electrolyte disturbances rather than the coma which are dangerous to life. Bleeding may occur, especially from the gastro-intestinal tract, due to the irritant action of the salicylate on mucous membranes, and from interference with the action of prothrombin. Occasionally sudden death may occur before coma or dyspnoea has developed; this may be due to hypersensitivity to the drug, small amounts producing a fatal reaction.

Diagnosis. The symptoms may be misleading, as the overbreathing, with ketosis due to dehydration, may suggest diabetic or uraemic coma. On other occasions the patient may initially appear normal, in spite of being severely poisoned. Urine containing salicylate will give a purple colour with a phenistix strip (Ames).

Laboratory Tests. Determination of the blood level of salicylate is very important as an indicator of the severity of poisoning; when an overdose has been taken it will be over 30 mg per 100 ml. Blood electrolytes and p^H should also be determined, especially in children, in whom salicylate poisoning is especially dangerous.

Treatment. Gastric lavage is usually indicated, since

much aspirin may be unabsorbed. Bicarbonate increases the excretion of salicylate in the urine, and so some should be left in the stomach, but beware of producing alkalosis. Forced alkaline diuresis has been especially recommended and haemodialysis may be necessary in severe cases. Otherwise correction of electrolyte disturbance and dehydration, together with general symptomatic measures, is required.

Autopsy findings. The stomach will usually contain a mass of white gritty powder, with inflammation of the lining and the presence of altered blood. The only other likely findings are multiple purpuric haemorrhages on the viscera.

Paracetamol

Another readily available analgesic drug, this is increasingly used in suicidal attempts. Poisoning is likely to occur with amounts of about 10 G. Nausea and vomiting is usually succeeded by evidence of liver damage, which may amount to total necrosis, and prove rapidly fatal. Renal damage may also occur. Gastric lavage, if the patient is seen soon after taking the drug, and supportive treatment for the liver failure is indicated.

CHAPTER 26
Corrosives

General aspects

All corrosive poisons have in common, as their principal characteristic, chemical damage of tissues coming directly into contact with the poison. Many of them have additional systemic effects, to be considered under the various individual poisons, but their main symptoms and lines of treatment can be considered as a group.

Sites of action (figure 22 a–d)

These substances are mainly colourless liquids, and are either swallowed or splash the skin. The sites likely to be affected by local contact and the principal effects are summarised in figure 22.

Main lines of treatment are:

Early. 1 Pain—treat with morphine, local anaesthetics, etc.
2 Dehydration—swallowing usually impossible, therefore I.V. fluids.
3 Corrosion—prevent further damage by neutralising poison.
4 Oedema of glottis—tracheotomy.
5 Gastric lavage—debatable, may remove poison, but may perforate stomach. If much damage probably better avoided.
Later. 6 Oxygen, antibiotics for pulmonary oedema or infection.
7 Surgery for perforations and later for stenoses.
Obviously emesis should be avoided in treatment because of the risks of perforating the stomach or spilling corrosive into the air passages.

Individual poisons

Sulphuric Acid (Part 2 Poisons List) (Lethal dose 1 oz = 30 ml)

One of the strongest corrosives. Usually an industrial or laboratory hazard, from concentrated acid, but battery acid

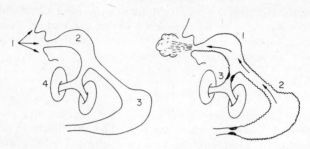

(a) Sites of action
1 Skin face or elsewhere
2 Mouth and throat
3 Upper alimentary tract
4 Respiratory tract

(b) Early effects
1 Pain and shock
2 Vomiting
3 Respiratory obstruction
  from laryngeal oedema

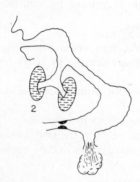

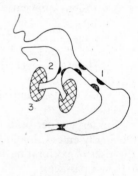

(c) Later effects
1 Perforation of stomach
2 Pulmonary oedema or
  bronchopneumonia

(d) Late effects
1 Oesophageal or pyloric
  stenosis
2 Laryngeal stenosis
3 Pulmonary fibrosis

Fig. 22

(30%) is strong enough to cause poisoning. The acid extracts water, produces heat and chars and blackens tissues. It should be neutralised with magnesia or soapy water. Avoid bicarbonate as sudden production of CO_2 could rupture the stomach. It is also known as oil of vitriol and used to be thrown at enemies to cause disfigurement. The crime of vitriol throwing is still a felony. More recently it has been used to destroy the bodies of murder victims (Haigh).

Hydrochloric Acid (Part 2 Poisons List) (Lethal dose 30 ml)

The effects are similar but slightly milder than sulphuric acid. The irritant fumes may cause the predominant symptoms to be respiratory, e.g. cough, dyspnoea and respiratory obstruction. The skin is not burnt.

Nitric Acid (Part 2 Poisons List) (Lethal dose 30 ml)

The effects are similar to those of the other acids but the stains and corrosion have a yellow colour. Nitrous fumes from acid are very dangerous (see later p. 243).

Hydrofluoric Acid (Lethal dose 4–5 G of fluoride)

Together with fluoride salts this substance is principally used in industry, but may be used as a rat poison. Symptoms of poisoning are of severe gastro-intestinal corrosion, and may be associated with the effects of lowered blood calcium, e.g. tetany, muscle cramps, bradycardia, etc. Contact with the skin may cause severe devitalising burns.

Acetic Acid (Lethal dose 60–70 ml)

Similar in effects to other acids. The smell is diagnostic. Irritation is the principal effect, corrosion less severe than with the mineral acids.

H

Caustic Alkalis (Part 2 Poisons List)

Caustic soda (NaOH) or caustic potash (KOH).

These have similar effects to the mineral acids, but the damaged tissue has a slimy feel, and is grey brown in colour at first, becoming blackened later.

Neutralisation is with dilute acids, the most readily available usually being vinegar.

Ammonia (Lethal dose—uncertain, 30 ml or less)

Most of the few cases of alkali poisoning which occur each year are with this substance. The circumstances may be those of suicide, but accidental poisoning occurs in industry, or when elderly persons with no sense of smell drink cleaning fluid containing ammonia.

Ammonia is a corrosive liquid with intensely irritating fumes. Therefore either the alimentary or the respiratory system may be principally affected.

If inhaled, the fumes may cause sudden cardiac inhibition and death, or after a period of coughing and choking, followed by a quiescent period, tracheo-bronchitis or pneumonia may develop. The ammonia vapour is particularly dangerous because it dissolves in the mucus of the air passages, and so its action is prolonged.

If ingested, the usual symptoms of corrosive poisoning are likely to develop. At autopsy the tissues are blackened due to the formation of alkaline haematin.

Treatment consists of neutralising with vinegar, and symptomatic measures. The initial prognosis must be cautious because of the insidious effect on the respiratory system.

Oxalic Acid (in Part 1, salts in Part 2 Poisons List) (Lethal dose about 15 G)

This substance has important systemic as well as local effects.

It is an uncommon cause of poisoning but the substance may occur at home or in industry as it is used for removing stains. Its local action, if concentrated, is corrosive to mucous membranes though not to the skin. Systemically it produces hypocalcaemia, and renal tubular damage, even in dilute solution.

The signs of poisoning will depend, therefore, on whether a large concentrated dose or a smaller dilute dose has been taken.

Large concentrated doses may cause sudden death by shock within a few minutes of ingestion. More often they produce the usual signs of corrosive poisoning, followed later by the systemic effects of hypocalcaemia and anuria.

Dilute doses will not have the corrosive effect. They may give some signs of gastro-intestinal disturbance, followed in a few hours by signs of hypocalcaemia, e.g. tetany, brady-cardia, etc. Within a few days signs of renal damage, oliguria and anuria may develop.

The initial treatment is gastric lavage, with neutralisation of the oxalate by calcium salts such as lime water. Symptomatic measures, possibly including haemo-dialysis, may be necessary.

Phenol (Part 1 of Poisons List) (Lethal dose about 10 G)

This substance also combines local and systemic effects. Locally grey-white corrosion which is anaesthetic is produced. Phenol can be readily absorbed through the skin.

If ingested the poison causes corrosion of the alimentary tract, though with little pain, and if inhaled laryngeal and pulmonary oedema are likely to result.

Systemically, phenol acts as a fat-soluble CNS depressant, like many anaesthetic agents, and so may produce sudden collapse and coma with respiratory depression. This may occur whether absorption is through the alimentary tract, respiratory tract or skin. Treatment is symptomatic. It is important to treat skin contamination by washing and to remember the danger of inhalation of fumes from any spilt phenol.

Paraquat

With the ready availability of this herbicide, cases of poisoning have started to increase. Taken as a liquid or granules, it produces initial symptoms of corrosion of the upper gastro-intestinal tract, with ulceration of the tongue. After a few days a progressive and untreatable acute pulmonary fibrosis begins, leading to death from respiratory failure.

CHAPTER 27

Coma—Cerebral Depressants

At the present time a victim of poisoning who is deeply comatose when first seen, is most likely to be suffering from the effects of an overdose of a barbiturate (see Chapter 25). The drugs described in this chapter are less commonly responsible for poisoning, but also are likely to present with coma as their principal symptom.

Narcotics

Morphine

Poisoning by morphine produces a deep coma, with contracted 'pin-point' pupils, very slow respiration (about six/ minute), warm sweating skin, and hypotension. Excretion of urine is diminished, and reflexes depressed.

With large doses death may occur from respiratory depression within an hour, but with smaller amounts coma is likely to be prolonged with the risk of hypostatic pneumonia occurring.

The lethal dose is about 180 mg, but children are disproportionately sensitive to the drug, for their body size.

Treatment consists of maintenance of respiration, often by artificial means, and the injection of the specific antagonist nalorphine, 5–10 mg I.V. every two hours, up to a total of 40 mg. This substance competes with morphine for the tissue receptors. The stomach should be washed out with a 1/2000 solution of potassium permanganate, to oxidise the drug. Excretion is mainly in the urine, and therefore the bladder should be emptied by catheter.

Morphine is a component of chlorodyne (with chloroform), laudanum (tincture of opium) and paregoric (camphorated tincture of opium), so that overdoses of these substances will produce morphine poisoning. Opium (from poppy heads) will also produce the same picture, but is ten times less toxic than morphine.

Heroin, dihydrocodeine, methadone and omnopon (papaverine) have similar effects.

Pethidine

This is a synthetic drug, which is mainly metabolised in the body, not excreted. It is an excellent analgesic but its hypnotic effect is only slight, compared to morphine; instead it tends to have a cerebral excitatory effect, and an overdose will initially have similar effects to atropine or cocaine, i.e. flushed face with dilated pupils, dry mouth, tachycardia, pyrexia, vomiting, excitement, tremors and convulsions. These may be followed by coma, and death from respiratory depression. The fatal dose is about 2 G.

Much smaller doses can produce alarming, and even fatal collapse if the drug is given at the same time as a monoamine oxidase inhibitor or a phenothiazine drug.

Treatment of the coma should be as for morphine, but with particular care in the use of any analeptics for fear of exaggerating the excitatory effect of pethidine and precipitating convulsions.

Chloral

Although a reliable hypnotic, overdoses of the order of 2–10 G may be fatal, with deep coma, and failure of peripheral circulation, and respiration. Gastric irritation may cause vomiting in the early stages. Other commonly used hypnotics which may cause death from deep cerebral depression are carbromal, Welldorm (dichlorphenazone), Doriden (glutethimide) and Mandrax (methaqualone).

Paraldehyde

Although a valuable hypnotic this drug may also produce cerebral depression and coma in overdosage, e.g. 25 ml (1 oz) by mouth. An alternative hazard is the conversion of some of the drug, during storage, to acetic acid, with the production of corrosion and acidosis when administered.

Quinine

This is freely available as tablets, and as a constituent of tonic mixtures. Often used as an abortifacient. Derived from bark of the cinchona tree.

It is a gastric irritant, causing nausea and vomiting, which is rapidly absorbed. It acts as a cerebral depressant, with particular action on cranial nerves. Thus early signs are headache, tinnitus and blurred vision followed by convulsions and coma. If the patient recovers consciousness she may be permanently blind, or deaf, or both. Haemolysis and haemoglobinuria may also occur.

Death may occur from respiratory paralysis during coma,

or later from anuria due to blockage of renal tubules by the products of haemolysis.

The toxic dose is probably of the order of 8 G.

Treatment consists of a gastric lavage and symptomatic measures are required. Blindness can be prevented in some cases by treatment designed to dilate the retinal vessels, such as stellate ganglion blockage, or the use of drugs such as amyl nitrite or nicotinic acid.

Chloroquine, which is used as an anti-malarial drug, and which has been consumed accidentally, or with intent to procure abortion, may, in overdosage, produce collapse, and death within a short time from sudden cardiac arrest.

Antihistamines

Source. Obtainable as tablets and capsules for use in allergic states and for the prevention of travel sickness.

There are no restrictions on sale, therefore freely available, and particularly dangerous for small children.

Effects. In adults the drugs exert a sedative effect which may be dangerous if the drugs are taken by drivers of motor vehicles, etc. Overdosage will cause the prompt onset of coma, with respiratory depression.

In children poisoning may produce cerebral excitation with restlessness and muscle twitching progressing to convulsions, followed by coma with respiratory depression and cerebral oedema.

Treatment. Gastric lavage and symptomatic measures, e.g. the use of sedatives to control convulsions.

CHAPTER 28
Convulsions—Cerebral Stimulants

A great many poisons can produce convulsions at some stage
of their effects. This may occur during the earlier stages of
cerebral depression, even though the principal effect of the
substance is to produce coma, e.g. barbiturates, carbon
monoxide and antihistamines, and resembles the excitation
which occurs during the early stages of anaesthesia. The
drugs described below have as their main effect the production of cerebral stimulation, usually with convulsions,
although at the later stages of poisoning exhaustion and
cerebral depression may occur, with coma, and death from
respiratory depression.

Strychnine

Source. Derived from the seeds of an Indian tree. There
are various injections and mixtures containing the salts,
hydrochloride, nitrate and sulphate. It was used to effect
homicidal poisoning in the nineteenth century, but is nowadays only likely to be encountered in circumstances of
accidental poisoning from overdoses of various tonic mixtures which contain strychnine, or from vermin poisons.
Children are especially at risk, from tonic preparations, e.g.
Easton's Tablets, left in accessible situations by adults.

Effects. It causes stimulation of the CNS, especially the
spinal cord, with exaggeration of reflex arcs. The fatal dose
is about 60 mg. Effects commence within about 15 minutes
of absorption, and are first apparent as twitching of muscles
and the complaint of a feeling of stiffness. This is soon
followed by a generalised convulsion, affecting all voluntary

muscles of the body. Contraction of the back extensors produces opisthotonus, the hands are clenched, the face distorted into a 'grin'. Spasm of intercostal and diaphragmatic muscles causes respiratory paralysis and cyanosis. Consciousness is retained and intense pain experienced. After about one minute the spasm relaxes, and is replaced by exhaustion and respiratory depression. Death may occur after two or more fits. There are no characteristic signs on the body after death, or detectable at autopsy. Differential diagnosis from tetanus may be difficult, but the latter usually has a more insidious onset, a history of injury, affects jaw muscles particularly, and muscles remain tense between spasms.

Treatment. The urgent need is to control the muscle spasms by the use of sedatives such as a barbiturate given intravenously, or paraldehyde, or by anaesthesia, and by muscle relaxants such as curare or gallamine.

Once such control has been achieved it may be necessary to maintain respiration artificially. The stomach should be washed out, using a dilute (1/2000) solution of potassium permanganate.

Amphetamine

Source. Amphetamine and similar drugs (dextramphetamine, methyl amphetamine, etc.), used medically for the treatment of obesity by reducing appetite, and to produce cerebral stimulation when combined with other drugs such as barbiturates. They were widely used as drugs of addiction, but a voluntary ban on their prescription, by doctors and pharmacists, has reduced this.

Effects. Overdosage may cause cerebral excitation with continuous purposeless physical activity, raised blood pressure, and hyperpyrexia. Hallucinations and convulsions may progress to exhaustion and coma with respiratory paralysis. The lethal dose is uncertain, but is of the order of 300 mg.

Treatment. The principal treatment is sedation to control the cerebral excitation by barbiturates or chlorpromazine, and symptomatic measures to reduce hyperpyrexia.

Cocaine

Source. Derived from the leaves of a South American tree, it is used in medicine to a limited extent nowadays as a local anaesthetic, for surface application only. Addicts use the powdered drug as a snuff and this may cause nasal ulceration.

Effects. Its medical value lies in the production of local anaesthesia, with which is coupled a vaso-constrictor effect. Systemically it rapidly produces stimulation of the cerebral cortex, followed by depression. The toxic dose is probably of the order of 1 G.

Even normal doses may produce sudden collapse and death in susceptible individuals. Poisoning by a large dose causes cerebral stimulation with excitement and confusion progressing to convulsions which are followed by coma, with respiratory depression and death. The pupils are dilated, and the victim may complain of a sensation of insects crawling over the body (formication).

Treatment. By control of excitement by short-acting barbiturates, and maintenance of respiration, and by gastric lavage with dilute potassium permanganate or charcoal.

Local anaesthetics

Many of these have toxic effects similar to cocaine, especially procaine, amethocaine, cinchocaine and lignocaine. Sudden cardiovascular collapse and death is relatively more common than cerebral excitement, and may occur during minor therapeutic procedures, such as bronchoscopy or pudendal block. Local anaesthetic solutions may contain adrenaline, which in overdosage may also have a toxic effect.

Atropine

Source. Accidental poisoning may occur from medicines containing atropine, e.g. from liniments, from belladonna plasters by absorption through intact or ulcerated skin, the ingestion of eye-drops or liniment, etc. Children may eat the berries of deadly nightshade (*Atropa belladonna*). Sufficient of the drug may be absorbed from the installation of eye-drops to produce bizarre symptoms on occasion.

Effect. Produces CNS stimulation and parasympathetic post-ganglionic blockade.
Pnemonic:
1   Hot as a hare—pyrexia of 1 to 6°F.
2   Blind as a bat—dilated fixed pupils—no near focus and temporary blindness.
3   Dry as a bone—suppression of salivation, as well as other secretions.
4   Red as a beet—vasodilatation and scarlatiniform erythema.
5   Mad as a hen—restless and agitated, hallucinations, delirium, incoordinated staggering gait, and incoherent speech.
The lethal dose is about 100–150 mg for adults.

Treatment. If the poison was ingested gastric lavage is indicated, though if children have eaten berries, then emesis may be preferable as the berries will probably not pass through the stomach tube. The physiological antidote is a parasympathomimetic drug, i.e. physostigmine 1 mg or pilocarpine. Otherwise general measures should be employed, e.g. sedation, control of pyrexia, catheterisation for retention of urine, etc.

At autopsy evidence of poisoning is unlikely unless, in a child, berries are found in the stomach.

CHAPTER 29
Poisons producing Paralysis

Many metallic poisons such as lead or thallium may produce slowly developing peripheral neuritis with paralysis. The substances described here, however, are those which cause rapid and fatal paralysis, and among them are the most lethal of all the poisons.

Nicotine

Source. This is mainly found as insecticide solutions which may contain up to 98% of nicotine, but accidental poisoning can occur, especially in children, from swallowing tobacco or the tarry fluid which accumulates in pipes. The solution can be absorbed through intact skin, e.g. from contaminated clothing.

Effects. The substance behaves like curare in that it paralyses voluntary muscles, particularly the muscles of respiration, and blocks the nicotinic actions of the sympathetic and parasympathetic ganglia. Symptoms of poisoning may be an exaggeration of the effects of heavy smoking, e.g. nausea and vomiting, cold sweats, faintness and dizziness, and these may be followed by convulsions or coma, and respiratory paralysis.

If large doses are taken in a suicidal attempt, however, the victim is likely to collapse and die almost immediately from respiratory paralysis. A fatal dose may be about 60 mg.

Chronic poisoning may produce Buerger's disease (thromboangiitis obliterans) or tobacco amblyopia.

Treatment. Any contaminated clothing must be removed at once, and skin washed.

Ingested poison may be removed by gastric lavage with dilute potassium permanganate.

Since the main lethal effect of nicotine is respiratory paralysis, principally of the muscles, but in heavy doses of the medulla also, and since the substance is rapidly destroyed in the body, artificial respiration until the effects of the poison have worn off is the most important measure in saving life.

At autopsy the stomach may be stained brown and smell of stale tobacco.

Cyanide

Sources. Solid sodium and potassium cyanides are used in industrial processes, and are readily available for use in various hobbies, e.g. photography. Hydrogen cyanide gas is used for fumigation. Liquid hydrogen cyanide (Prussic Acid) is used in industry and by veterinary surgeons and is an ingredient of certain medicines.

Effects. Cyanide inhibits the oxidising enzyme, cytochrome oxidase, and prevents the uptake of oxygen by the cells.

As a result the blood remains fully oxygenated, so that both arterial and venous blood have a uniform bright red colour. The lethal amount of Prussic Acid is about 2 ml, and of alkaline cyanide about 300 mg.

The consumption of such a quantity of cyanide is often followed by collapse and death within seconds, but on occasions death may be delayed for many minutes, the victim being in deep coma with almost undetectable pulse and respiration, and in such cases the specific treatment may save the victim's life.

Treatment. This is one of the few poisons where a specific antidote is really important in treatment, and when available, should precede all other measures. The antidotes used are nitrites and sodium thiosulphate. Nitrites form methae-moglobin which then combines avidly with cyanide to form cyanmethaemoglobin. The thiosulphate combines with cyanide to yield thiocyanate.

Speed is essential when applying these measures. First the patient must be kept breathing by artificial respiration, and inhalations of amyl nitrate given, while the other antidotes are being prepared. These are 0·3 G sodium nitrate in 10 ml water, followed by 25 G of sodium thiosulphate in 50 ml of water, given slowly (over 10 minutes) intravenously.

After the antidotes have been given the stomach should be washed out. The antidotes may be repeated after 1 hour. Very recently success has been reported by treatment with Cobalt E.D.T.A.

Autopsy findings. The bitter-almond smell of cyanide may be apparent at the scene of death or when examining the body, but many people are unable to detect the odour. The hypostasis may be bright red, due to the oxygenated blood, but the appearance can be confused with carbon monoxide poisoning or exposure of the body to cold.

Internally, the organs will also be bright red in colour. Sodium or potassium cyanide may degenerate with time to produce ammonia and sodium or potassium hydroxide, therefore poisoning with these substances may produce the signs of corrosive poisoning in the alimentary tract, and may cause the stomach to smell of ammonia.

Organo-phosphorus compounds

Source. These substances are used in agriculture as insecti-cides in the form of sprays or dusts. The compound which is best known as a poison is Parathion, which is common as a suicidal or homicidal poison on the Continent, but in this country the only cases reported have been accidental. There are many similar compounds, e.g. TEPP, Malathion, etc., though most are much less toxic than Parathion.

Effects. The poison may be absorbed through intact skin, inhaled, or ingested. It acts by inhibition of cholinesterase enzymes, so that acetyl choline accumulates at nerve endings, producing stimulation, then paralysis, especially of voluntary muscles. Parathion is extremely toxic and an oral dose of 200 mg may be fatal. Because of this, extensive protective measures are taken, e.g. protective clothing, etc., when the substance is used industrially.

Large overdoses may produce immediate death.

Smaller doses cause nausea, vomiting, sweating abdominal colic, contracted pupils and muscle twitching, followed by convulsions and coma, with muscular paralysis and death from respiratory failure.

Treatment. Contaminated skin must be cleansed and respiration maintained. Specific antidotes are atropine 2 mg hourly together with P.A.M. (2 pyridine aldoxine methiodide) or pralidoxime chloride 15–30 mg/kg body weight.

At autopsy there are no distinctive features of the poison itself but it is commonly supplied in a solvent, such as paraffin, and this may impart a distinctive odour to the tissues.

T.O.C.P. (Tri-ortho-cresyl Phosphate)

Source. An oily liquid, it is used in lubricants and as a plasticiser in industry. Mass outbreaks of poisoning have occurred from contamination of food by containers which previously held the poison. The abortifacient, apiol, may be contaminated by this substance.

Effects. The poison is said to inhibit pseudocholinesterase enzymes with resultant damage to myelin nerve-sheaths. Soon after swallowing the poison there is a transient gastric upset. This is followed by a latent period of several days' duration, after which pains in the back and legs develop followed by flaccid paralysis of the muscles. The condition may be mistaken for poliomyelitis or some other type of peripheral neuritis.

Aconite

Source. This is derived from the plant *Aconitium rapellus* or Monkshood, which is grown in many English gardens. It is a component of some medicines, notably liniment ABC.

Effects. The poison is extremely dangerous, 2 mg of the active principle, aconitine, being said to constitute a fatal dose. The action of the alkaloid is on nerve endings, and, to a lesser extent, on the brain.

If swallowed there is an initial tingling of the lips and mouth, followed by vomiting and dysphagia. A sensation of coldness extends over the body with progressive muscular paralysis, the pulse rate is slowed and death results from respiratory paralysis.

Conium (Hemlock)

Derived from the hemlock plant, found throughout Britain. The alkaloid coniine has an action resembling that of curare, with progressive motor paralysis extending upwards from the extremities until death results from respiratory paralysis. The drug was used to poison Socrates. Treatment is by artificial respiration, oxygen, analeptics, etc.

CHAPTER 30
Inebriants

For the clinical diagnosis of drunkenness, see Chapter 11.

Ethyl alcohol

In addition to the various alcoholic drinks, beers, wines, spirits, etc., alcohol is also available as a laboratory reagent and as surgical or industrial spirit.

Effects. Its action in producing drunkenness by paralysis of the higher centres in the brain is described in Chapter 11. It acts as a cerebral depressant in a similar manner to an anaesthetic agent. When small amounts of alcohol are present in the body the depressant action is masked by the euphoric effect of the release of lower cerebral centres but with larger amounts depression becomes apparent, as inco-ordination develops, followed by coma. At very high blood levels, 400–500 mg per 100 ml, medullary paralysis with failure of respiration will occur. Asphyxia from inhalation of vomit, or injuries sustained during intoxication may also cause death.

Treatment. A drunken patient who is unconscious needs the same care in diagnosis and treatment as does any other victim of poisoning. He requires skilled observation and a careful differential diagnosis of the condition from other causes of coma, notably head injury. Deeply unconscious persons may need gastric lavage, maintenance of a clear airway, and intravenous glucose, or fructose, and possibly analeptics, oxygen and assisted respiration.

At autopsy the body is likely to smell of alcohol. The stomach may be congested, possibly with acute erosions. The air passages may contain vomit. The possible coincidence of poisoning by other drugs must be remembered.

In the case of chronic alcoholism, the liver may show gross fatty change, or lobular cirrhosis, sometimes associated with oesophageal varices. There may be evidence of vitamin deficiencies, or malnutrition and the heart can develop an alcoholic cardiomyopathy. The ultimate cause of death is likely to be an infection.

Methyl alcohol

Source. Pure methyl alcohol is used in industry or as an antifreeze substance. In the form of methylated spirit it is mixed with ethyl alcohol, pyridine, and methyl violet. 'Meths' drinkers may be found in the vagrant community of any city, in conditions of extreme social degradation. The pyridine may give their skin a distinctive purple colour.

Effects. Methyl alcohol produces drunkenness as does ethyl alcohol, but with certain distinct differences due to the fact that metabolism of the alcohol is slow, most being excreted unchanged, and the remainder oxidised to formic acid. The effects are partly due to a direct toxic action of the methyl alcohol, but mainly to acidosis. As a result:

1 The effects are delayed, often for 24–36 hours, unless very large amounts have been taken, and early symptoms may be masked by the coincident absorption of ethyl alcohol.

2 Nausea and vomiting are associated with abdominal pain.

3 Eye signs—headache, photophobia, followed by blindness.

4 Acidosis—with rapid respiration, ketonuria, etc.

5 In heavy overdosage prolonged coma may lead to death from respiratory paralysis in 12–24 hours, or more.

Treatment. Cautious administration of ethyl alcohol may prevent oxidation of methyl alcohol and so reduce the development of acidosis.

Acidosis must be treated with sodium bicarbonate, or sodium lactate intravenously. Large amounts of fluid should be given. Morphine may be needed for pain. Gastric lavage should be performed using a solution of sodium bicarbonate.

Antabuse (Disulphiram)

This is a drug which is used in the treatment of chronic alcoholism to produce cure by aversion. Death has occurred when a person taking antabuse has consumed a large amount of alcohol, as the amount of aldehyde formed (the drug prevents oxidisation of alcohol beyond the stage of aldehyde formation) has reached lethal levels, with cardiovascular collapse.

Antifreeze-Ethylene Glycol

Poisoning has occurred when this substance has been consumed accidentally. It has also been used as a substitute for alcohol, especially by soldiers, or in under-developed countries.

In the early stages cerebral symptoms are produced; later, if the patient survives, renal damage may occur. The early symptoms are drowsiness, progressing to coma, and are frequently mistaken for drunkenness. If recovery from this phase occurs, symptoms of renal damage, oliguria or anuria, may occur a few days later.

An autopsy there is evidence of nephosis, with typical fan-shaped crystals in the renal tubules.

Methyl Pentynol (Oblivon)

As a liquid or in capsules this is used as a mild sedative, e.g.

before dental extractions. It is an alcohol, and combined with other drugs, such as barbiturates, may produce additive effects.

Cannabis indica

Source. Also known as hashish or indian hemp and marijuana in America, it is derived from a plant grown in India and China, and occasionally in fine summers in this country. Import is illegal, as the drug is a potent source of addiction, but the drug is smuggled into this country. It is taken in the form of cigarettes.

Effects. Stage of intoxication—the symptoms are of mild intoxication with pleasant hallucinations, sexual excitation, etc.

Stage of narcosis—larger amounts cause dizziness and atoxia, delirium, then deep sleep. A fatal outcome is rare but may occur from respiratory failure. 2 g of the drug may be fatal.

Treatment is by analeptics and assisted respiration.

The main danger of hashish is not of fatal poisoning, but of the progression of the addict to more potent and dangerous drugs of addiction (see Chapter 36).

CHAPTER 31
Irritants—Metals

Among these substances are some of the most notorious homicidal poisons, e.g. arsenic and yellow phosphorus.

Nowadays they are chiefly of importance as industrial hazards, but their use is sufficiently widespread to lead to occasional poisoning in domestic circumstances.

Acute poisoning. Any of these substances are likely to present with similar features, i.e. thirst; metallic or burning taste; abdominal pain; vomiting: diarrhoea; dehydration and circulatory collapse, and possibly death. Treatment is along general lines—gastric lavage, analgesics, I.V. fluids, warmth, etc., but there are specific antidotes for some of the metals. The features of chronic poisoning vary according to the poison responsible (see below).

Lead

Source. This metal can cause unsuspected poisoning as it can be derived from many different sources, e.g. in water which has passed through lead pipes, or in alcohol prepared or stored in vessels with a lead glaze, or from the use of battery casings for fuel, and in children who chew paint or toys which contain lead, apart from industrial processes. Poisoning is occasionally due to the accidental ingestion of soluble lead salts. Lead can also be inhaled, and absorbed through broken skin (e.g. lead lotion compresses).

Effects. Acute poisoning, e.g. from drinking lead acetate solution, has the typical features of irritant poisoning but rarely proves fatal.

Chronic poisoning. Small amounts of lead (e.g. 0·5 mg/day) are constantly being absorbed from the environment, so that a healthy person will normally have traces of lead in his tissues, but accumulation is prevented by excretion in urine (0·05 mg per litre/day) and faeces, such that a balance is maintained between ingestion and excretion.

In health the amount of lead in the blood does not exceed 0·08 mg per 100 ml.

In chronic poisoning excessive amounts are absorbed and cannot be excreted so that lead accumulates in the tissues, especially in the liver, kidneys and bones. The blood level rises above 0·08 mg and may reach 1·0 mg per 100 ml.

The symptoms of chronic poisoning are:

General	pallor, loss of weight
	anorexia and a metallic taste
	abdominal colic—relieved by pressure
	constipation
	blue line on gums
Cardiovas-cular	vaso-constriction, causing pallor and hypertension
	rarely hypertensive encephalopathy
Renal	albuminuria, chronic nephritis
Locomotor	interference with the enzymes involved in muscle contraction, therefore muscle weakness develops especially in the muscles most used, e.g. wrist-drop.
Blood	hypochromic anaemia, due to mild haemolysis and defects of haemopoesis; punctuate basophilia.

Diagnosis. (a) Clinically—History of exposure. Constipation, with abdominal pain, pallor, normal pulse, muscle paralysis, blue line on gums.

(b) Laboratory (i) urine—more than 0·08 mg lead per litre urine (24-hour samples are necessary). (ii) blood—0·08 mg lead per 100 cc blood.

The containers for the samples must be lead-free. Certain types of glass or plastic may contain traces of lead.

Treatment. Gastric lavage—in acute poisoning, with sodium or magnesium sulphate to precipitate insoluble lead sulphate and cause purgation.

The specific treatment to remove lead from the tissues is by the use of chelating agents, e.g. EDTA (ethylene diamine tetra-acetic acid), administered by the slow I.V.

infusion of 0·5–1 G per 30 lb body weight per day, or penicillamine, orally, 750–1500 mg/day.

Lead poisoning in children (see Chapter 35)

Lead poisoning in children is likely to present as an encephalopathy and has a poor prognosis. Chronic lead poisoning is thought to be responsible for some cases of mental deficiency.

Tetra-ethyl lead poisoning

This compound is used as an additive in petrol. Poisoning may occur in garage workers. Early symptoms of insomnia and mental changes may lead on to delirium and mania, and death may occur from exhaustion.

Mercury

Sources. Principally an industrial poison, the metal is used in the manufacture of thermometers, explosives, etc. Mercuric chloride may be used as a disinfectant. Mercurous compounds have been used in teething powders. Organic mercury compounds are used as diuretics, and alkyl compounds as seed dressings.

Effects. Mercury may be absorbed by various routes:
1 The skin—from lotions, or the innunction of metallic mercury.
2 Ingestion—accidental swallowing of corrosive sublimate, the use of some teething powders which contain mercury, etc.
3 From the vagina, bladder, or rectum—from the use of mercury compounds as douches or antiseptic lotions.
4 Inhalation—mercury evaporates slowly at room temperature, and so the air above a pool of mercury may contain appreciable amounts of the metal.

The action of the poison by combining with sulphydryl groups is to inhibit the action of certain enzymes. Excretion is via the kidneys, large bowel and salivary glands, and thus these organs are particularly affected by poisoning.

Acute poisoning

E.g. from swallowing corrosive sublimate, 1 g likely to be fatal. Severe irritant symptoms occur, together with salivation and persistent diarrhoea, and one or two days later nephrosis and anuria may develop.

Chronic poisoning

Usually occurs from industrial exposure.

Symptoms. 1. *Ptyalism*—persistent salivation and infection of the mouth and gums with loosening of the teeth.

2 *Tremor*—coarse and jerky, of small muscles such as those of the hands. The condition was once known as 'Hatter's Shakes', from the use of mercury in the fur felting industry.

3 *Erethism*—emotional disturbances, e.g. irritability, with insomnia and excessive timidity or anger.

4 *Renal damage*—nephrosis and uraemia.

General effects—emaciation, gastro-intestinal disorders, etc.

Special forms of poisoning

Alkyl mercury poisoning—from eating treated seeds or from the vapour. The main effects are on the nervous system, with ataxia and dysarthria and restriction of visual fields. Large outbreaks have occurred in some under-developed countries.

Pink disease—acrodynia occurs in young children, from mercury compounds, notably in teething powders. The children are miserable, with muscle weakness and skin rashes, and reddening of the hands and feet.

Mercurial diuretics—intravenous injection has caused sudden collapse and death.

Treatment

Acute poisoning requires gastric lavage. Egg albumin will precipitate the poison and must then be removed by lavage. Anuria will require appropriate treatment. The specific antidote for acute or chronic mercury poisoning is BAL, given as 5 mg/kilo initially, then half as much at 4-hourly intervals. Penicillamine has also been found of value. Symptomatic treatment will be necessary.

Arsenic

Sources. The most notorious of the homicidal poisons, restrictions ensure nowadays that the principal source of the poison is in industry, such as in glass manufacture, sheep dips, fruit sprays, etc. Traces occur naturally in some soils, well waters, shellfish, etc. Mass poisonings have occurred occasionally from accidental contamination of food. The various forms of arsenic which cause poisoning are arsenious oxide, various arsenites and sulphites of arsenic, arsine gas, and organic arsenicals.

The lethal dose of arsenious oxide is about 120 mg. The principal effects of poisoning are produced by combination of the poison with sulphydryl groups of enzymes.

Symptoms. 1 Ingested poison. (a) *Fulminating*—massive doses may cause shock with peripheral vascular collapse and death may occur in 1 or 2 hours. This form of poisoning is rare.

(b) *Acute*—the typical effects of irritant poisoning are

produced, i.e. pain, vomiting, diarrhoea, circulatory failure. Death may occur in 12–36 hours.

(c) *Chronic*—when taken in small doses over a period of weeks or months. General debility, weight loss, chronic gastro-intestinal disturbance, mental irritability, loss of hair, 'rain-drop' pigmentation of the skin and hyperkeratosis of palms and soles, and peripheral neuritis.

2   Inhaled poison. Arsine gas AsH_3, is an industrial hazard. It produces massive haemolysis. Death may occur at once, or within a few days, due to renal damage resulting principally from the effects of haemolysis.

3   Injected poison. Organic arsenicals, e.g. used in treatment of syphilis, have produced sudden collapse and death. The overuse of pessaries containing arsenic, e.g. for trichomonas, has also caused poisoning.

Laboratory Tests. Arsenic may be found in the stomach contents in cases of acute poisoning, and in blood and urine, faeces, and hair of cases of chronic poisoning.

After burial arsenic may remain detectable in the organs for many months and the body tends to be abnormally well preserved. Care must be taken to exclude the possibility of contamination of the body by arsenic derived from the soil of the grave before arriving at the conclusion that death was due to poisoning.

Treatment. Acute cases—gastric lavage. If available ferric hydroxide will precipitate any poison remaining in the stomach. The specific antidote is BAL, which has greater affinity than the sulphydryl groups of the enzymes for arsenic. It should be given as early as possible in an initial dose of 3 mg per kilo body weight, then half this amount at 4-hourly intervals for 36 to 48 hours.

In chronic poisoning the patient must be removed from the source of poisoning, and treatment with BAL instituted.

Antimony

This substance is similar in many respects to arsenic. It is used in tropical medicine, and in industry. The compounds mainly responsible for poisoning are potassium antimony tartrate (tartar emetic) and antimony chloride. It has been used for homicide, but toxic effects are nowadays likely to be the result of accidental ingestion. Group poisonings have occurred from contamination of food and drink by traces of antimony in the enamel of utensils. It does not occur naturally in soil.

The effects are similar to those of arsenic, i.e. blockage of sulphydryl groups. The lethal dose is about 1 G. Vomiting is particularly pronounced (hence tartar *emetic*). Antimony may damage the heart muscle and cause bradycardia or sudden heart failure, especially when given intravenously as in the treatment of tropical diseases.

Treatment is by gastric lavage and BAL. Tannic acid, e.g. strong tea, may precipitate any poison remaining in the stomach.

Phosphorus

When phosphorus was a constituent of rat poisons, and therefore readily available to the public, cases of poisoning were not infrequent in this country. Now its only source is likely to be in industry. There are two forms of phosphorus, the yellow, which is poisonous, and the red which is innocuous. The lethal dose is about 300 mg.

Effects. The poison has a garlic odour and taste, and is unlikely to be taken accidentally. It can produce 3 forms of poisoning.

(a) *Fulminating.* Death occurs in a few hours, and the principal features are of peripheral vascular collapse.

(b) *Acute.* The most common form. Initial symptoms are of irritant poison, burning pain, vomiting, severe thirst. The vomit may be luminous. These symptoms last for up to 48 hours. Then for one or two days there is a remission of symptoms. Finally signs of liver damage develop, with enlargement of the liver, jaundice, multiple haemorrhages and hepatic coma.

(c) *Chronic.* This form of poisoning is rare, but has occurred in workers handling phosphorus, poisoning being from the fumes. The principal effect is necrosis of the bones of the jaws, together with chronic gastro-intestinal disturbances and liver damage.

Treatment. Gastric lavage with dilute potassium permanganate to oxidise the phosphorus, and general measures for shock, liver failure, etc.

Copper sulphate will neutralise the phosphorus and a copper sulphate-soap mixture is useful in the treatment of phosphorus burns of the skin, which are deep and devitalising. It must not, of course, be given systemically as it is itself poisonous.

At the autopsy of a person who has died in the early stages of poisoning, signs of acute gastro-intestinal irritation with luminous garlic-smelling intestinal contents are indicative of the poison. If the victim has survived for a few days, jaundice with acute fatty changes or necrosis of the liver and fatty degeneration of other organs, together with multiple haemorrhages within the body, are likely to be found. When taking samples it must be remembered that elemental phosphorus will be rapidly oxidised if the material is exposed to air for any time and so samples must be put into sealed containers as soon as possible. The stomach and bowel are better left unopened.

Thallium

As yet a rare poison in this country; its use as a depilatory in the treatment of ringworm was discontinued in 1930. Abroad it is a constituent of rat pastes, and has been used as a homicidal poison, for which its properties are almost ideal.

It produces abdominal pain and vomiting, after a delay of 12–24 hours. The illness continues over the next two or three weeks with peripheral neuritis, cerebral symptoms, disturbances of sleep, and a rash, and death may occur from respiratory or cardiac failure. The most striking symptom is the sudden and almost total loss of body hair.

Barium

Barium sulphate, as used in X-ray examinations, is harmless, but barium carbonate or chloride are toxic, and so poisoning may occur from the mistaken use of the wrong substance, or from accidental contamination of food, e.g. by flour containing barium sulphate, prepared as a rat poison.

The symptoms are of gastro-intestinal irritation, i.e. pain and vomiting, and of stimulation followed by paralysis of muscle fibres with muscle twitching and convulsions followed by respiratory and cardiac arrest.

Chromium

Chronic poisoning in industry produces ulcers in the skin and nasal septum (chrome holes). Ingestion of chromates causes severe gastro-intestinal irritation, followed by kidney damage and anuria.

Cadmium

The danger is chiefly from the inhalation of the fumes.

These have a necrotising action on alveolar membranes, with severe pulmonary oedema, followed, if the victim survives, by pulmonary fibrosis.

Beryllium

This substance produces chronic granulomas, if inhaled or introduced into the skin through cuts. Severe pulmonary fibrosis can result.

Zinc

Inhalation of fumes can cause inflammation of the lungs and bronchopneumonia. Ingestion of zinc sulphate or chloride will cause intense gastro-intestinal irritation, and possibly corrosion.

CHAPTER 32
Poisonous Gases and Hydrocarbons

Carbon Monoxide

Source. Until recently all domestic gas supplies contained CO. Now the gradual introduction of natural gas is reducing the amount of carbon monoxide present. It is also produced by incomplete combustion due to a restricted supply of air, e.g. a lighted paraffin heater in an unventilated room. It is an important cause of death in burning buildings.

Effects. The gas is absorbed rapidly through the lungs into the blood where it is taken up by haemoglobin in preference to oxygen, producing carboxyhaemoglobin. As this process continues, less and less haemoglobin remains available to transport oxygen, and death results from anoxia.

Lethal Dose. Conversion of more than 50% of the haemo-globin to carboxyhaemoglobin will cause death. In the elderly, or in persons suffering from some serious disease, 30% to 40% conversion may be fatal.

The time taken to die will obviously depend on the concentration of gas inhaled. Thus if pure carbon monoxide is absorbed, as in laboratory accidents, two breaths will absorb sufficient gas to prove fatal. Domestic supplies contain about 4% of carbon monoxide, and inhalation may continue for 15–20 minutes before death occurs, and even longer if the gas is diluted by air in a well-ventilated room.

Signs of poisoning. Cerebral anoxia will cause coma, possibly preceded by convulsions. The carboxyhaemoglobin has a characteristic bright pink colour, which can be seen in the nail beds, the lips, etc. At autopsy the hypostasis, and the internal organs will have the same colour.

Laboratory Tests. Carboxyhaemoglobin has a characteristic spectrum by which it can be identified, and, using a Hartridge reversion spectroscope, the amount present in the blood can be determined. Various chemical methods are also available.

Treatment. This consists of removing the victim from the contaminated atmosphere, and administering oxygen and assisting respiration if the person is severely poisoned. The anoxia may cause myocardial damage, so that complete rest is necessary for several days. Cerebral anoxia may lead to neurological sequelae.

Circumstances. These are almost always either accidental, e.g. in elderly persons who do not smell escaping gas from unlit appliances or people using heaters with inadequate ventilation, or suicidal, usually indicated by the presence of suicidal notes, and such preparations as the provision by the deceased of mattresses to lie on and the arrangement of towels, cushions, etc., to seal off air leaks round doors and windows.

However, when examining the scene of death the doctor should always bear in mind the possibility of murder, the body having been arranged subsequently so as to make the scene appear to be one of suicidal gassing.

Chlorine Cl_2

Although principally an industrial hazard, poisoning has occasionally occurred in domestic circumstances by liberation of chlorine from lavatory cleansers.

The gas produces inflammation of the lungs and pulmonary oedema, and if the victim survives pulmonary fibrosis may result. Some elderly chronic bronchitics owe their present disability to chlorine poisoning sustained in the First World War.

Phosgene $COCl_2$

In addition to industrial sources, it may be produced from the action of heat on carbon tetrachloride and trichlorethylene, and thus can be a hazard of the use of some fire extinguishers in confined spaces.

Initial irritation of the respiratory tract, with coughing and choking, is followed, after a latent interval of a few hours, by intense pulmonary oedema. Characteristically at autopsy there is little inflammation of bronchial mucous membrane, in spite of the pulmonary oedema, a finding which distinguishes poisoning by this substance from the effects of chlorine.

Hydrogen Sulphide H_2S

This gas is produced by putrefaction and so may be found in sewers and tunnels, as well as being produced by various processes in the chemical industry.

The concentrated gas produces fatal poisoning within a

few minutes, and lower concentration may cause prolonged unconsciousness, due to cerebral depression.

Sulphur Dioxide SO_2

Responsible for much of the effects of polluted city air on those with respiratory trouble, it may in high concentration cause severe oedema of the larynx or bronchospasm. Being used at high temperatures in some industrial processes, it may cause burns, which have a characteristic appearance due to fixation instead of charring of thè tissues.

Carbon Disulphide CS_2

Used in many industrial processes. In high concentration it causes cerebral depression and coma, and may lead to respiratory failure. Chronic poisoning with cerebral symptoms, parkinsonism, chorea, peripheral neuritis, may occur.

Nitrous Fumes NO_2 and N_2O_4

Hazards of industry, and of laboratory accidents and fires, these red-brown irritating fumes produce initial coughing, followed by a latent interval, during which the patient appears to have recovered. However this interval is followed by the development of intense pulmonary oedema. Therefore it is dangerous to send home a person who has recently been exposed to these fumes, even if he appears well. He should be kept under observation for 24 hr, until the danger of pulmonary oedema has passed.

Carbon Dioxide CO_2

The effects of CO_2 retention in various diseases and in anaesthesia are well known. Pure CO_2 may cause immediate collapse and death, and is a hazard of coal-mining. It may also accumulate in wells, manholes, etc., and cause the

I

sudden death of workmen, often with further deaths among would-be rescuers.

Arsine see Arsenic

Phosphine PH₃

Smells like rotting fish, and is produced in various processes in the chemical industry. A highly toxic gas, it produces the symptoms of cholinesterase inhibition, resembling poisoning by Parathion (p. 225), i.e. salivation, sweating, colic, diarrhoea, convulsions, coma, with pin-point pupils, and death from respiratory depression.

Hydrogen Cyanide see Cyanide (p. 223)

Methyl Bromide CH₃Br

Used in fire extinguishers and as an insecticide. Very danger-ous when used in confined spaces. Symptoms of poison-ing are likely to be delayed for several hours, and then commence with gastric upset. The action on the central nervous system produces symptoms resembling mild intoxi-cation, ataxia, diplopia, etc., which are followed by convul-sions and pulmonary oedema. Renal tubular necrosis may develop.

Laboratory determination of the blood bromine level may confirm the diagnosis.

There is no antidote, treatment being by symptomatic measures.

Carbon Tetrachloride CCl₄

Used principally as a fire extinguisher or dry-cleaning agent, and as such it is found in many homes.

Poisoning can be due to inhalation of fumes, as when

using a fire extinguisher, or cleaning clothes in a confined space, or by accidental ingestion. Addiction to the fumes may occur, even in children. Coincident ingestion of alcohol increases the toxic effect of the poison.

Inhalations may produce rapid anaesthesia and death within a few minutes. Evidence of poisoning at autopsy is slight, but the organs usually have an odour of carbon tetrachloride, notably the brain, but this may be fleeting, and easily overlooked.

Ingestion of the poison causes initial gastric upset, followed by a latent period of a day or so, after which liver necrosis and renal tubular necrosis develop.

When used as a fire extinguisher, phosgene may be produced (see p. 242).

Tetrachlorethane $(CHCl_2)_2$

This solvent has many industrial uses. If swallowed accidentally or with suicidal intent it produces cerebral depression and, after a few hours, respiratory failure. Prolonged inhalation, as in industry, may cause fatty degeneration and necrosis of the liver.

Trichlorethylene—Trilene C_2HCl_3

Well known as an anaesthetic agent, and also having industrial uses, addiction to the vapour can occur among anaesthetists or workmen. Death has resulted in industry or among addicts from anaesthesia with cerebral and respiratory depression.

Petrol and Paraffin

Petrol is moderately toxic if swallowed. Inhalation of the fumes produces symptoms ranging from apparent drunkenness to coma and death within minutes, depending on the concentration of the fumes. Paraffin is particularly dangerous for children, who are likely to drink it. It may cause vomiting, and coma, but the principal danger is to the respiratory tract. Because of its low surface tension it can spread rapidly over the surface of bronchial mucous membranes and into the alveolar tree with widespread collapse of lung tissue. Symptoms are of dyspnoea, cough and cyanosis, followed by bronchopneumonia. X-ray films may show widely scattered opacities in the lung fields. If the child survives, severe pulmonary fibrosis may result.

As a consequence of the ability of paraffin to spread over mucous membranes it is one of the few poisons where gastric lavage is specifically contra-indicated, because of the danger of soiling the upper respiratory tract. Treatment is by oxygen and antibiotics.

CHAPTER 33
Poisons causing Methaemoglobinaemia

The poisons in this section, although chemically dissimilar, are grouped together because they have in common the function of producing methaemoglobin, which is likely to be their most immediately obvious symptom.

Methaemoglobin has a characteristic spectrum with one band in the red region. It does not form a loose complex with oxygen as does haemoglobin. Therefore the capacity of the blood to transport oxygen is reduced, and cyanosis and anoxia result. A characteristic 'slaty' appearance of the skin is produced, due partly to cyanosis and partly to the brown colour of the blood which is produced by methaemoglobin.

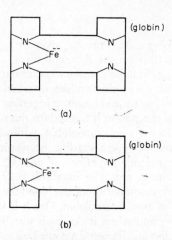

FIG. 23. (a) *Haemoglobin. The iron is in the reduced (ferrous) state. This combines loosely with oxygen. (b) Methaemoglobin. The iron is in the oxidised (ferric) state.*

Treatment

This consists of the reduction of ferric to ferrous iron, converting methaemoglobin to ordinary haemoglobin. The substance used is methylene blue. Usually this acts as an oxidising agent, and therefore would produce more methaemoglobin. But in low concentration in the body it is reduced by an enzyme to the colourless leuco-form, and then acts as a reducing agent, converting the iron in the blood from the ferric to the ferrous state.

The principal substances which will produce methaemoglobin are: aniline, nitrobenzene, nitrites, acetanilide, bromates, chlorates, pyrogallol,

These have other unrelated actions which are described below.

Aniline

Used in marking inks, crayons, dyes and polishes. It is easily absorbed through the skin, and this is the usual route of poisoning, e.g. in babies whose nappies have been freshly marked with ink containing aniline, or when aniline is spilt on a seat. Poisoning by inhalation or ingestion rarely occurs.

The effect of the poison is to produce the sudden onset of cyanosis, due to the methoemoglobin, without dyspnoea or other symptoms of severe cardiac or respiratory disease. Adults may experience the effects of anoxia, e.g. throbbing headache, dizziness, etc. The diagnosis may be confirmed by spectroscopic examination of the blood for the characteristic spectrum of methaemoglobin. Death is very rare, even in small babies, and when it occurs is usually due to associated disease, the anoxia being a contributory factor.

Treatment is by intravenous injections of methylene blue—the dose being 1–2 mg/kilo of body weight. Gastric lavage is necessary if the poison has been ingested, and in severe cases, oxygen may be required.

Nitrobenzene

This is an oil, known as oil of mirbane, which has an odour of bitter almonds. It is used in shoe and furniture polishes, lacquers, marking inks, perfumes, etc. Poisoning is usually from accidental ingestion, or may be by inhalation of the fumes or absorbtion through the skin. It is a more dangerous poison than aniline; death has resulted from about 1 G.

Symptoms, the onset of which may be delayed for several hours, consist of nausea and vomiting, with cyanosis due to methaemoglobinaemia. Severe poisoning may in addition cause symptoms of cerebral depression, with drowsiness and convulsions followed by coma. Death may occur from respiratory failure.

The diagnosis should be suggested by the smell of almonds about the patient, the cyanosis, often almost black, the chocolate-brown colour of a blood sample and its characteristic spectrum.

Treatment is by gastric lavage, intravenous methylene blue, oxygen, etc., and in a few cases haemolytic anaemia renders transfusion necessary.

Nitrites

Nitrites may be taken in error for common salt, etc., or ingested with suicidal intention. In country districts water derived from certain wells may contain organic nitrates which when ingested are converted by bacteria in the bowel to nitrites, which are then absorbed and cause poisoning.

The victims may present with apparently symptomless cyanosis, due to methaemoglobin.

Large doses of nitrites, as when taken with suicidal intent, may cause sudden collapse due to hypotension from dilatation of blood vessels, and death may occur almost immediately. 2 G may prove fatal.

Acetanilide and Phenacetin

Both these substances in common use as analgesics and antipyretics, may, with prolonged use, produce methaemoglobin, possibly by the release of traces of aniline within the body.

The prolonged use of phenacetin has also been found to produce chronic renal damage, notably interstitial fibrosis and papillary necrosis.Haemolytic anaemia may also occur. Sale of phenacetin is now prohibited, if the quantity is more than 0·1% except on prescription.

Chlorates

Sodium and potassium chlorate are occasionally used in medicine as gargles and for local oral application. Sodium chlorate is also obtainable as a weedkiller, and, being explosive when heated with oxidisable substances, is used in the match industry.

Poisoning usually occurs either from excessive use of medicinal preparations, or from the accidental consumption of weedkiller. 5 G in children or 10 G in adults may prove fatal.

Symptoms:

1 Gastro-intestinal upset—abdominal pain, vomiting, diarrhoea.

2 Blood—rapid and massive haemolysis, with production of Heinz bodies in red blood cells and the formation of methaemoglobin.

3 Renal damage—renal tubular obstruction following haemolysis with oliguria and anuria.

4 Hyperkalaemia—cardiovascular collapse.

Death may occur from circulatory failure, from anoxia, or from uraemia. A distinctive feature, at autopsy, is likely to be the chocolate-brown colour of the blood.

Treatment consists of gastric lavage, replacement of haemolysed blood by transfusion, and management of anuria.

Pyrogallol

Used in photography, hair dyes, ointments, etc. It can be absorbed through the skin. It produces gastro-intestinal irritation, with nausea and vomiting and methaemoglobinaemia.

CHAPTER 34
Miscellaneous Poisons

Bromides

Acute poisoning from these sedatives is very rare unless massive overdoses are taken. On the other hand chronic poisoning can occur easily, from prolonged consumption of therapeutic doses. The bromide replaces chloride in the blood and tissues, and so will accumulate slowly.

The symptoms develop insidiously and may easily not be recognised, being considered to be due to progression of the condition for which the sedative has been given. They consist of progressive dulling of the mental faculties with tremor and clumsiness and loss of memory, and of conjunctivitis with an acneform pustular rash. Ultimately mania, hallucinations, coma and death may occur.

The diagnosis can easily be confirmed by laboratory estimation of the blood bromine levels, toxic changes occurring when the level exceeds 150 mg per 100 ml.

Treatment is by sedation if confusion or mania is present, withdrawal of the source of bromide, and the administration of large amounts of water and chlorides, to displace the bromide from the tissues.

Potassium Permanganate

Although used in gastric lavage as an antidote, notably for narcotic poisons, it must be remembered that concentrated solutions of this substance will damage the tissues by oxidation. Any solution more concentrated than 1/1000 will cause injury, and for gastric lavage only solutions of 1/5000 strength or less should be used.

The substance acts as a mild corrosive. For this reason it has been used as an abortifacient, by douching with concentrated solutions or by the vaginal application of tablets of permanganate. Local ulceration results with profuse haemorrhage. The condition may be mistaken for an inevitable abortion and therapeutic measures appropriate to the latter condition instituted.

If swallowed the effects are of a corrosive poison. The lethal dose is of the order of 10–20 G. The diagnosis is suggested by the brown staining of the tissues. Rarely symptoms of hyperkalaemia may occur from absorption of the potassium ion.

D.N.O.C. (Di-nitro-ortho-cresol)

Principally used as weedkiller and insecticide. At one time it had a therapeutic use in the treatment of obesity.

Absorption can be through the skin, as well as by injection and inhalation, so that persons spraying crops are at risk if they do not wear protective clothing.

The action of the poison is to produce a considerable increase of the basal metabolic rate. Initial feelings of unusual well-being are followed by fatigue, insomnia, thirst and sweating, and loss of weight. Raised respiration rate and hyperpyrexia are followed by convulsions, coma and death.

There is no specific antidote. Treatment must be by sedation, reduction of pyrexia, rest, etc.

CHAPTER 35
Poisoning in Childhood

Poisoning of children is particularly important since they are more liable to suffer from accidental poisoning than adults, being prone to experiment with tastes and to put things in their mouths, and to be attracted by brightly coloured pills which resemble sweets.

The principle of diagnosis and treatment of poisoning in childhood is on the same general lines as adults, and no attempt is made, therefore, in this book to deal with the particular aspects of medical treatment of children, which are the province of pediatrics. Suffice it to say that poisoning should always be considered as a possible cause of sudden illness in a child, though the differentiation of such a condition from the early symptoms of an acute infection may be difficult.

Since accidental poisoning in children is so often preventable, doctors should endeavour whenever possible to ensure that parents lock medicines and poisons in safe places, out of the reach of children, and to avoid the accumulation in the house of large amounts of unused medicines.

The substances commonly causing poisoning in children are mostly those which are freely available and which also cause adult poisoning. These have been mentioned in detail in the preceding pages. A few substances however are likely to be especially consumed by children, or have peculiar dangers for them, and these are described in this chapter.

The principal substances causing poisoning in children are:

1   Salicylates.
2   Tranquillisers.

3   Iron preparations.
4   Barbiturates.
5   Strychnine.
6   Antihistamines.
7   Borax.

Others of importance, though less commonly responsible for poisoning, are:

8   Amphetamine.
9   Paraffin.
10 Lead.
11 Camphorated oil.
12 Digitalis.
13 Atropine.
14 Paraquat.

Salicylates (see p. 206)

Aspirin tablets or methyl salicylate liniment are equally dangerous. Thus 1 teaspoon of the liniment contains 45 gr of salicylate.

Poisoning may occur from accidental consumption of the ubiquitous aspirin tablets, but it may also occur from the excessive administration by parents of aspirin to children who are ill from some cause, such as a mild infection or from teething. The classical symptoms, e.g. dyspnoea, will be seen and the condition may be mistaken for pneumonia. Children are much more likely to die from salicylate poisoning than are adults.

Tranquillisers (see p. 213)

Reported cases have shown ataxia, nystagmus, athetoid movements and epileptiform convulsions, together with irregularities of the heart due to interference with the mechanism of conduction and with the risk of cardiac arrest.

Iron preparations

These are peculiarly dangerous for children, and the brightly coloured tablets may closely resemble sweets. A fatal dose may be 15–20 gr (i.e. 5–7 tablets).

Symptoms may occur in 3 stages:

1   Stage of gastro-intestinal irritation lasting about 6 hours, with abdominal pain, vomiting and shock due to necrotising effect of iron on the bowel mucosa.

2   Latent period, lasting about 24 hours, during which time the child appears to be recovering, though toxic products are being formed within the body.

3   Relapse due to development of acidosis. There may be convulsions or coma, with liver damage, and haemorrhages. Death may occur in either the first or third stage.

Treatment is by emesis to remove the tablets, or gastric lavage with sodium bicarbonate solution to precipitate the iron in the stomach. The specific antidote is desferrioxamine, some being instilled into the stomach (3–7 G in 50–200 ml of water) and some given by I.V. infusion in a dose of 15 mg per kilo body weight per hour, up to a total of 80 mg per kilo.

Antihistamines (see p. 217)

Children are more likely to be poisoned by these drugs than are adults, since only a small amount may constitute a toxic dose, e.g. 6 gr, and because antihistamine preparations are readily available in many homes being used as remedies for travel sickness or hay-fever.

The principal symptoms in children are likely to be of cerebral irritation with ataxia and delirium, followed by convulsions. Death may occur from respiratory depression.

Borax

This has been a common household substance used in the

care of children for many years, in the form of dusting powders or boracic lotion. The B.M.A. has (1966) advised doctors not to prescribe boracic compounds and the Poisons Board has recommended that manufacturers should stop making preparations containing boric acid and borates for infants.

Borax can be absorbed by ingestion, or through broken skin (e.g. a nappy-rash) but not through intact skin. Symptoms are:

Gastro-intestinal irritation—vomiting, diarrhoea, shock.

Rash—red and beefy.

Cerebral symptoms—delirium, convulsions and coma, with neck retraction (meningeal irritation).

Renal symptoms—oliguria and anuria.

The coincidence of gastro-intestinal and meningeal symptoms in a child with a pronounced skin rash should always suggest the possibility of borax poisoning.

Lead

Children are especially at risk from this particular substance. Sources of poisoning may be from the use of battery cases as household fuel, from lead toys, lead paints on cots, lead nipple shields used by the mother, etc.

Affected children will at first be listless, pale, and anaemic. However, unlike adults suffering from lead poisoning, the symptoms are likely to progress to the development of behaviour disturbances and restlessness, followed by encephalopathy, which may be fatal or cause residual mental retardation. Some cases of mental deficiency have been found to be associated with high levels of lead in the body.

Camphor

Poisoning is likely to be by the liniment, camphorated oil. Camphor was popular in medicine at one time as an analeptic, and so the symptoms of overdosage are of cerebral irritation, headache, restlessness and confusion, muscle twitching and convulsions. Poisoning is rarely fatal but may cause death from respiratory failure. A teaspoonful of the liniment may prove fatal to an infant.

Digitalis

From swallowing adults' pills or medicines. The effects of the poison are to produce nausea and vomiting, followed by cardiac disturbances, bradycardia, heart block, etc., as in overdosage in adults. Death from heart failure is rare.

Poisonous plants

Many common plants are poisonous and children are especially liable to eat their berries or chew their leaves. Some plants have already been mentioned—monkshood (aconite, p. 226), hemlock (conium, p. 236), foxglove (digitalis, p. 257), deadly nightshade (atropine, p. 221). Other plants commonly found which can produce poisoning, usually with gastro-intestinal irritation as the principal feature, are laburnum, broom, privet, daphne mezereum, cyclamen, hawthorn, horsechestnut.

Similar danger may arise from toadstools. The most dangerous is *Amanita phalloides*, the Death Cap. Effects are delayed for several hours, when vomiting, abdominal pain and diarrhoea commence and become severe, with dehydration and shock. After 3 or 4 days liver or renal failure is likely to develop, with coma and death.

Other mushrooms, e.g. *Amanita muscaria*, may produce symptoms suggesting alcoholic intoxication, with salivation, nausea and vomiting, hallucinations and convulsions.

CHAPTER 36

Drug Addiction

At one time a minor problem in this country, with addiction confined to the morphine group of drugs and with addicts only numbered in a few hundreds, the situation has altered rapidly in recent years. It is considered that there are nowadays large numbers of persons addicted to drugs of many different types, sedatives, stimulants, etc., as well as the narcotics, and such addiction is increasingly found among young persons, even schoolchildren.

With a view to dealing with these problems, the Drugs (Prevention of Misuse) Act of 1964, and the Dangerous Drugs Act 1965 and 1967 were enacted. These have now all been superseded by the Misuse of Drugs Act 1971. Under the provisions of the last-named statute, a doctor will be required to notify to the appropriate authority particulars of any person who he suspects is addicted to drugs. He may not supply drugs to such persons except under licence from the Home Secretary, and contravention of regulations made under the provisions of this Act may result in the doctor being prohibited from supplying such drugs of addiction. Alleged contravention of regulations by doctors may be considered by special tribunals. For further details see Chapter 9.

Certain groups of drugs are especially prone to produce addiction, and this danger must be borne in mind when prescribing such drugs for a patient.

Morphine group

These were the original and are the best-known drugs of addiction, principally opium, morphine, pethedine, heroin, methadone, etc. They produce intense craving and severe withdrawal symptoms, and heroin especially is associated with rapid physical and mental degeneration. Treatment of a patient by one of these drugs for more than two weeks is liable to produce addiction. The drugs are frequently self-administered intravenously, with lack of sterile precautions, and so addicts may be recognised by thrombosis of superficial veins and multiple small abscesses at injection sites on arms and legs. Apart from the general physical and moral effects of addiction, the victims are also at risk of overdose of the drug, septicaemia and serum hepatitis. The drugs can be detected in the urine, as can most of the other drugs of abuse, except some of the hallucinogens.

Cocaine group

These produce intense craving for the drug, but no physical withdrawal symptoms. The drug is frequently taken as snuff, which has resulted in perforation of the nasal septum, and its use may precede addiction to drugs of the morphine group. The addict is likely to show excitement, and will probably experience 'formication', a sensation as of insects crawling under the skin.

Cannabis group

Cannabis does not usually cause physical deterioration or withdrawal symptoms, and addiction does not produce social degeneration caused by the other substances, but it is dangerous because it often acts as an introduction for young people to the other forms of addiction. Its symptoms are rather similar to alcoholic intoxication, and the drug is usually taken by inhalation from cigarettes ('reefers'). The smell of burning cannabis is characteristic.

Barbiturate group

Any barbiturate or any sedative drug can produce addiction,

the patient taking progressively larger amounts, much greater than the therapeutic dose. There may be severe withdrawal symptoms. Consumption of such a sedative for more than four weeks may produce addiction. These drugs may be taken together with alcohol, or with stimulant drugs, and in such circumstances may produce sudden and unexpected death. Though usually taken orally, they may be administered intravenously, with similar dangers to those described under morphine above. The starch excipient of the capsules may produce microemboli of the lungs, detectable at autopsy.

Amphetamine group

These drugs are particularly liable to be taken by young people for their stimulant action, though voluntary control of prescribing by doctors and pharmacists has considerably reduced the problem. Addicts may be restless, or experience paranoid hallucinations, have a dry mouth and ulceration of the oral mucosa and may develop sleeplessness, maniacal behaviour or even hyperpyrexia.

Hallucinogenic group

Although such drugs as LSD (Lisergic acid diethylamide), mescaline, etc., are not yet proved to produce true addiction, illegal supply has allowed them to reach the groups of society who are particularly liable to drug addiction. They have been responsible for several deaths, since they produce hallucinations in the recipients, with such impressions as that they could fly, dive through brick walls, etc. They can produce terrifying psychotic episodes. Many of the drugs are produced in illegal laboratories, and as the dose is very small, can be supplied in such vehicles as small pieces of paper impregnated with tiny drops of the solution.

Medical practitioners should always be on their guard to recognise addicts or potential addicts, to be cautious in prescribing any of the drugs known to produce addiction, and to ensure that large supplies of drugs are not available in patients' homes to be passed on to those without authority to receive them. The requirements of the Misuse of Drugs Act 1971 must be observed precisely, not least because failure to do so will render the doctor liable to prosecution.

Treatment of drug addiction should only be carried out by medical practitioners having special experience and facilities, e.g. in mental hospitals, and such treatment should not be undertaken lightly. The proposed centres to be set up by the Government may answer the problem of treatment. The prevention and cure of drug addiction is as serious a problem as prevention of the major infectious diseases, because of its terrible destructive effect on the physical well-being of the patients, and on their mental states. The drugs themselves are unlikely to cause criminal behaviour, except the stimulants and hallucinogens, but crime, robbery, prostitution, etc., are resorted to in order to obtain the funds with which to obtain further supplies of the drug, and addiction once established is very difficult to cure.

Index